I0832181

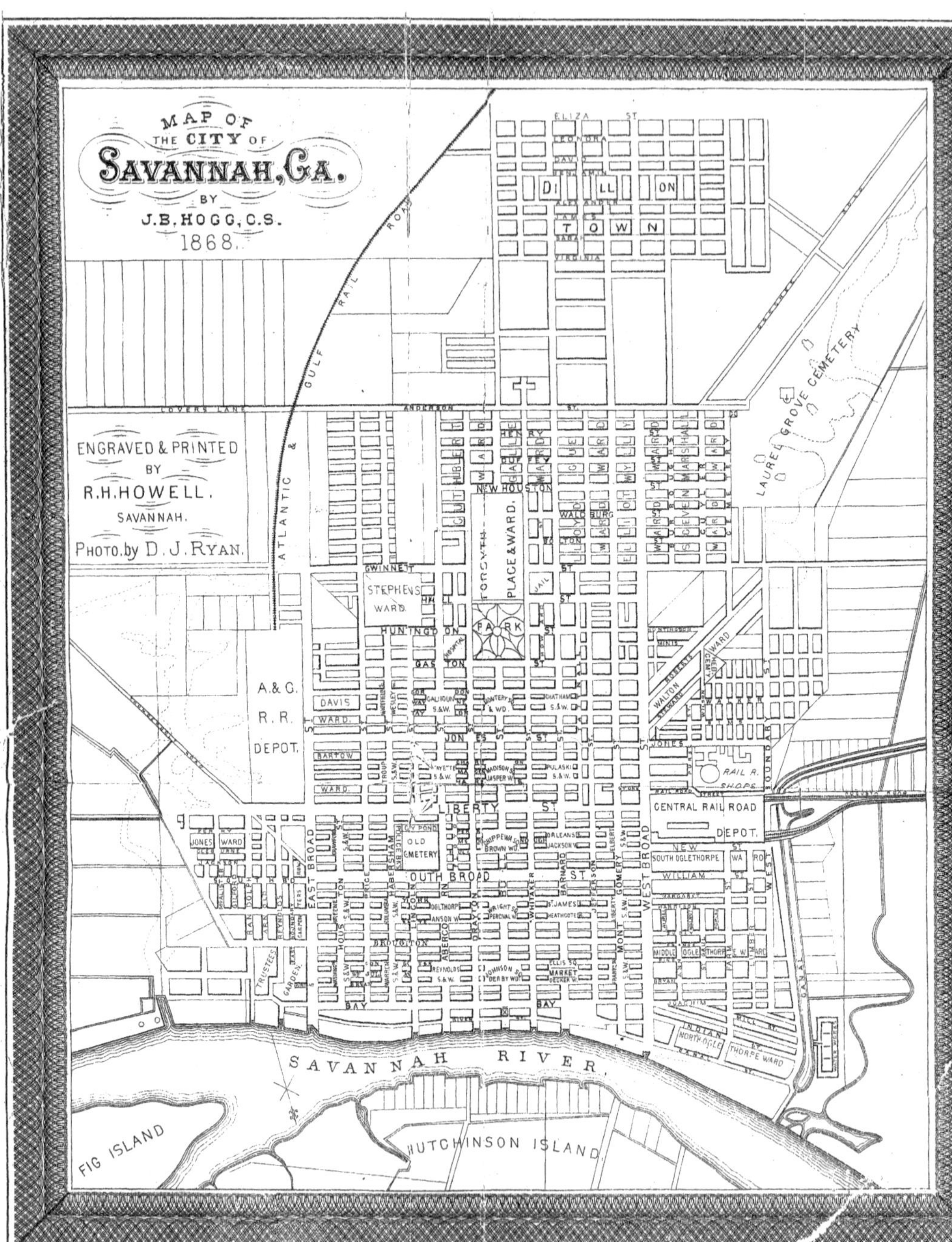
MAP OF
THE CITY OF
SAVANNAH, GA.
BY
J.B. HOGG, C.S.
1868.
ENGRAVED & PRINTED
BY
R.H. HOWELL.
SAVANNAH.
PHOTO. by D. J. RYAN.
DILLON
TOWN
LAUREL GROVE CEMETERY
ATLANTIC & GULF RAIL ROAD
ANDERSON ST.
LOVERS LANE
FORSYTH PLACE & WARD.
PARK
STEPHENS WARD.
A. & G. R.R. DEPOT.
DAVIS WARD.
BARTOW WARD.
JONES WARD
OLD CEMETERY
LIBERTY ST
SOUTH BROAD ST
EAST BROAD
WEST BROAD
CENTRAL RAIL ROAD DEPOT.
RAIL R. SHOPS
NEW SOUTH OGLETHORPE WARD
BAY
SAVANNAH RIVER
FIG ISLAND
HUTCHINSON ISLAND

HISTORICAL RECORD

OF THE

CITY OF SAVANNAH.

BY F. D. LEE AND J. L. AGNEW.

SAVANNAH:

PRINTED AND PUBLISHED BY J. H. ESTILL,

MORNING NEWS STEAM-POWER PRESS,

1869.

TO THE

BUSINESS MEN OF SAVANNAH,

WHO, FROM THE DAYS OF THE PIONEERS OF BUSINESS TO THE PRESENT TIME, DESPITE THE RUINOUS PROSTRATION OF TRADE AND COMMERCE, OCCASIONED BY

WARS, FIRES, GALES, AND PESTILENCE,

HAVE BROUGHT THEIR CITY TO THE PROUD POSITION SHE NOW HOLDS IN THE COMMERCIAL WORLD, THE

HISTORICAL RECORD OF SAVANNAH

IS RESPECTFULLY DEDICATED.

PREFACE.

"History," said that eminent writer, Lord Bolingbroke, "is philosophy teaching by example." If this assertion be true, either philosophy has been very select in her examples or history not very judicious in her selections or her teachings. Historians, until very recently, have only found illustrations of life and of fact, and examples for teaching philosophy, law, and morals, among Kings and Nobles, Warriors and Statesmen. The People, the foundation of the social fabric, with their interests and rights, their thoughts and feelings, their personal toils and domestic life, have only figured in general history as machines for Kings to use or weapons for warriors to employ—the one not caring how soon the machine wore out, the other quite as reckless of the waste of weapons. The pomp of royalty, the problems of philosophers, the shifts and subterfuges of statesmen, and the butcheries of warriors fill the panorama of the world's life as it moves along the pages of the historian. Even here the assertion, as the majority of historians exemplify it, contradicts the facts and teachings of all ages—that the history of the world, as the history of life, is made up of little things. After all that has been written of the eminent and mighty men of ancient and modern times, how little do we know of the inner, personal, and domestic life of communities and nations. Pompeii has revealed more to awaken thought and excite curiosity and disgust than all the histories of Rome from Remus to Pio Nono. A remark of Erasmus in a letter written by him to a friend concerning the domestic life of England in his time—stating that the floors of the houses are commonly of clay, strewed with rushes, under which lie unmolested a collection of beer, grease, fragments of meat, bones, spittle, excrements of dogs and cats, and of everything that is nauseous—throws more light upon the household civilization and social filthiness of the aristocracy than all the tomes of Hume in detailing the pomp and power, the pride and prowess of its Kings, its Statesmen, and its Warriors. Only think of the grand and queenly Elizabeth sitting on a leathern couch or straw pallet, making a breakfast of salt beef and brewer's beer? Or standing ankle-deep in filthy straw, pulling pieces of roasted ox into bits for her dinner and throwing the refuse to snarling dogs—new accretions from dainty hands to the sweltering mass of filth and putrescence already rotting upon the floor. Until Lord Macauley entered into these recesses of the inner social life of the former times in England very few of her population knew from what small and rude beginnings the present social civilization of their country had grown.

All civilization grows up from and out of small centres and humble sources. A man, a house, a settlement, a machine, are the starting points of new and grand developments of social life and national history. The world is full of such records that find illustration and culmination in the fame and wealth and power that give success and triumph to personal enterprise and stability and grandeur to a nation's history. These are the memorials of *the people*—the historic monuments lifting their heads in the sunlight and blazing from foundation to capstone with the effulgence that time and truth shed on the useful and the good. These, whether they come down from the dim and shadowy past or have their birth and fruition in the near and still remembered, are the antiquities of a place and a people. In the usual acceptation of the term, our country has no antiquities. Art, science, literature, music, poetry, war, have left no records, given us no monuments. Its physical character, its broad prairies, its long rolling rivers, its vast inland seas, its hidden and exhaustless mineral wealth, its grand old forests, its extensive coast line, its glorious and majestic mountains—these are its monuments; but they are monumental of "Eternal power and Godhead." Aside from these—and with these what do we lack for aught that wisdom can employ or skilful labor produce—our only antiquities are indian life and history, and the wreck and remnants of colonial times. The former, as to its origin and incidents, is involved in mystery and mixed with fable. But it is replete with interest to the curious and gorgeous with thrilling tales of field and flood to the workers of fiction. The latter blushes yet in virgin loveliness and beauty, and yet lifts its maiden hands, imploring Old Mortality to decipher its inscriptions, to freshen its facts, to revivify its memorials and hand down to the generations coming and to come "the short and simple annals" of the people who from holy religious principles and love of liberty settled the lands which their children have enriched as a garden and made to "bloom and blossom as the rose."

Jamestown, Croatan, Charleston, Savannah, are the colonial starting points of States that have given dignity and fame to American civilization and new elements of truth and power to augment the wealth of the world's history. These names and places, however waste and desolate some of them may now be, are monumental, and historic literature will keep them living and fresh in the memory of ages.

Of Jamestown, a portion of the tower of its first church and the grave-stones of its forgotten dead are all that time has left of its material history and physical and social fortunes. Croatan is the dwelling-place of a small population, who gain a scanty subsistence as pilots and fishermen. Charleston, judiciously located at the confluence of two rivers whose tides mingle and are lost in the rushing waves of the Atlantic, perpetuates the good sense of its first settlers. Savannah grew into a city beautiful for situation, the joy of a State and renowned among the cities of our land for its trade, commerce, industry, and enterprise, as well as for its intelligence, its wealth, and its refinement. Its history is a souvenir of truth and honor—a memorial of the sagacity and forethought that in February, 1733, selected it as the home of the English colonists, the site of a city that now graces the beautiful river on whose side it stands and whose name it bears. The philosophy of its foundation and fortunes belong to the examples and facts of history. The tents under the four pine trees on the bluff have grown into a city that looketh out over the sea and stretcheth its hands of trade to collect and transmit the wealth of the Empire State of the South. The indians, who greeted and gave a home to those comers from a land over "the great and wide sea," have given place to the guests they welcomed with strange words and uncouth ceremonial. Their wigwams no longer crown the bluff, they no longer paddle the light canoe over the flashing waters of the river; warrior and maiden, with their brave deeds and simple loves, chief and brave, council-tent and home, have all disappeared. A new day, a new people with the principles and powers of a new life, entered this wilderness when the small vessel, with Oglethorpe on its deck, passed in from the sea and sped its way up the placid river to the village-crowned bluff on its shore. The elegant and luxuriant mansions of the flower-crowned city of to-day are the consummation and glory of that "day of small things." Between these days one hundred and thirty-five years of history, civil and social, personal and domestic, unfold their pages of trial and triumph, progress and pause, toil and suffering, virtue and licentiousness, life and death. Art, science, trade, commerce, law, literature, festivals and fasts, religion and vice, all await, each with its contribution of glory or shame, to fill the measure of the city's history. The records are brimming full.

The object of the compilers is to open the long-closed volume, bring things long hidden out into the sunlight, make scenes long lying in darkness and shadow, names long lost amid passing events, voices long silent address us from the graves of the past; let us purchase, sit down and listen, "read, mark, and inwardly digest" the facts to be disclosed and the words to be spoken.

In placing this humble work before the public, the compilers would state that they claim nothing for it beyond what its name denotes—a brief record of the historical events connected with Savannah from the earliest period of its existence to the present time. They hope that it will be thorough, and constitute a standard book of reference to all who desire to inquire into the history of the city of Savannah. To obtain information necessary to complete this record, much difficulty was experienced, and in many instances it was impossible to gain the desired facts. Especially was it difficult to obtain the names of the soldiers of Savannah who served during the late war. Many of the rolls of companies could not be obtained, and we were compelled to rely upon scraps of rolls, and frequently upon the memories of a few soldiers who cheerfully gave us all assistance in their power. Many of the facts contained herein were condensed or excerpted from McCall's and Bishop Stevens' Histories of Georgia, White's Historical Collections of Georgia, Colonel C. C. Jones' Record of the Chatham Artillery, and from old records in the possession of the Georgia Historical Society and citizens. To those who have rendered us assistance we tender our grateful thanks.

CONTENTS.

CHAPTER I.

CHAPTER II.

CHAPTER III.

Chapter VI.

Chapter VII.

CHAPTER VIII.

SAVANNAH AS IT IS.

SAVANNAH.

> "I walk these ancient haunts with reverent tread,
> And seem to gaze upon the mighty dead;
> Imagination calls a noble train
> From dust and darkness back to life again."

One hundred and thirty-five years ago a small tribe of indians occupied the bluff upon which the city of Savannah now stands. Then the indian's canoe, only, ruffled the placid waters of the Savannah; now steam and sail vessels from every clime, attracted by the fruits of Savannah's commerce, plough its bosom, coming and going, with keels deeply sunk in the water. Then the smoke curled lazily upward from a few wigwams; now fiery furnaces belch forth volumes of ruddy flame, and on every hand is heard the din of hammers and bellows, the voices of men echoing from the manufactories, wharves, and places of business, where a numerous population are plying the tireless fingers of industry in the creation of substantial wealth. Then the woods resounded with the savage warwhoop; now the no less discordant, but more civilized, steam-whistle is heard as the heavily-laden trains pass to and fro on the iron arms which have been stretched in every direction, clasping in their embrace some of the choicest regions of the country. On every hand are elegant and luxurious mansions, gardens teeming with flowers of richest and rarest hue; churches and humane institutions; colleges and schools; squares and park thronged with mature and youthful beauty, making the balmy atmosphere vocal with sounds of human life and joy—all attesting wealth, refinement, piety, benevolence, intelligence, health, and happiness.

1

CHAPTER I.

Origin of the Settlement of Savannah — Departure of the Colonists — Their Arrival at Charleston — Oglethorpe's Visit to Yamacraw — Arrival of the Colonists on the Bluff — Friendly Overtures of the Indians — Oglethorpe's Description of Savannah — Kindness of South Carolinians — Treaty with the Indians — Arrival of the First Ship — Laying Out of the Town, and Naming of the Streets, Squares, Wards, and Tithings — Arrival of Hebrew Settlers — Alligators become Troublesome — Arrival of the Salzburgers — Oglethorpe Goes to England — Appearance of Savannah in 1734 — A Judge Acts in a Three-fold Capacity — Wine and Silk Culture — Discontentment — Arrival of Revs. John and Charles Wesley.

About the year 1729, the sufferings of the poor people of England, especially the debtors, who, by the laws of the country which gave to the creditor complete control over them, were thrown into prison, there to remain in rags and misery the rest of their days, enlisted the sympathy of a number of influential men of London, who visited the debtors' prisons and adopted measures for their relief. But owing to the existing laws very little good was accomplished, and they sought other means of relief.

These gentlemen, John Lord Viscount Percival, Edward Digby, George Carpenter, James Oglethorpe, George Heathcote, John Laroche, James Vernon, William Beletha, Stephen Hales, Thomas Tower, Robert More, Robert Hucks, Roger Holland, William Sloper, Francis Eyles, John Burton, Richard Bandy, Arthur Bradford, Samuel Smith, Adam Anderson, and Thomas Coram, petitioned the Throne to grant them a charter for a separate and distinct province from Carolina, between the Savannah and Altamaha rivers, to which they designed sending a number of poor people who had neither lands nor other means of supporting themselves and families.

On the ninth of June, 1732, his Majesty King George the Second granted the charter, in his letters-patent, reciting, among other things, "that many of his poor subjects were, through misfortunes and want of employment, reduced to great necessities, and would be glad to be settled in any of his Majesty's provinces in America, where, by cultivating the waste and desolate lands, they might not only gain a comfortable subsistence, but also strengthen his Majesty's colonies and increase the trade, navigation, and wealth of his

Majesty's realms; and that the province of North America had been frequently ravaged by indian enemies, more especially that of South Carolina, whose southern frontier continued unsettled and lay open to the neighboring savages; and to relieve the wants of said poor people, and to protect his Majesty's subjects in South Carolina, a regular colony of the said poor people should be settled and established on the southern frontiers of Carolina."

Acting under the authority of their charter, the Trustees held their first meeting in July, 1732, and made arrangements for carrying their designs into execution. Money was collected and persons selected to be sent over and settled in the new colony, which they resolved should be on the Savannah river. James Oglethorpe, who had been foremost in these philanthropic designs, resolved to accompany the colonists, and used every effort toward obtaining worthy persons. No lazy or immoral persons, none who would leave families, none who could obtain subsistence in England, and none who were in debt and could not obtain the consent of their creditors, were selected. By the 16th of November, 1732, thirty-five families, numbering in all about one hundred and twenty-five "sober, moral, and industrious persons," had been selected and embarked on the galley Ann, a vessel of two hundred tons burthen, commanded by Captain John Thomas, then lying in the Thames, a short distance below London. Here the Trustees visited them, and asked each family if they were satisfied and desired to go, giving them the privilege of remaining behind if they so wished. Only one man, who had left a sick wife at Southwark, declined to go. They then bid the colonists farewell, and on the following day, the 17th of November, the vessel sailed from Gravesend. Among the emigrants was Rev. Henry Herbert, D. D., who had volunteered to accompany and aid them without any compensation.

After a weary voyage, during which one delicate infant died, the vessel arrived in Rebellion Roads, at Charleston, and cast anchor, on the 13th of January, 1733. Oglethorpe immediately landed, and was hospitably received by Governor Johnson and the Council of South Carolina, by whose order the King's pilot carried the vessel into Port Royal, and on the 20th the Colonists were landed at Beaufort and lodged in the new barracks of his Majesty's Independent Company. The officers of the company, and the people of the town, bestowed every attention possible upon the new-comers.

Leaving the Colonists here to rest themselves and recover from the fatigue incident to their long voyage, Oglethorpe, accompanied by Colonel William Bull, of South Carolina, sailed in a small vessel to the Savannah river, to select a site for the proposed settlement. Arriving in the river, a pine-crowned bluff attracted their attention, and they landed to inspect it. They found on the western end of the bluff a little indian village called Yamacraw. The chief of the tribe to which the village belonged was named Tomichichi. In the village was a trading-house owned by a white man named John Musgrove, Jr., who had married a half-breed woman named Mary. She could speak both the Indian and English languages.

The top of the bluff was comparatively free from trees, level, and admirably adapted for the establishment of a settlement, and Oglethorpe being well pleased with it, appealed to Mary to obtain from the tribe permission for the emigrants to settle there. The tribe at first refused to grant the request, and threatened to "dig up the hatchet" if the settlers came. After much persuasion on the part of Mary, a provisional treaty was granted until the whole Creek nation could be consulted. Deeming this satisfactory, Oglethorpe selected the site, about the centre of the bluff, named it Savannah, after the river which flowed at its foot, secured the services of Mary as interpreter for the whites in subsequent intercourse with the indians, and left for Beaufort, arriving there on the 24th of January. Here he secured a sloop of seventy tons and five plantation boats, and on the 30th the colonists embarked for the bluff.

They arrived here on the first of February and landed on the western end of the bluff, that being the only point from which an ascent could be readily made. The tents and baggage were carried up the bluff and along it to four pine trees, under which the four large tents were pitched, one for each tithing, into which municipal divisions the colonists had been divided before their arrival.

The tents had scarcely been pitched, and the baggage and bedding placed therein, before the indians came to salute the colonists, from whose presence they expected to reap many benefits. In front of the king and queen, who were followed by about twenty of the tribe, came the "medicine-man," advancing with strange and uncouth antics, having in each hand a spread fan of white feathers, fastened to a rod, hung from top to bottom with little bells, with which he approached Oglethorpe (who had advanced a short distance from his tent to meet them), and related the deeds of their ancestors, all the while stroking him on each side with the fan, as an expression of the friendship of the tribe. The king and queen then welcomed the General, after which the indians partook of an entertainment prepared for them in the General's tent.

Work was the "order of the day" for several days after the landing, and, under the supervision of their leader, the men felled trees, hewed timber, cleared the land, and erected palisades. On the 9th, Oglethorpe and Colonel Bull marked out a square, the streets, and forty lots for houses, and on the same day commenced the first house.

The following day General Oglethorpe wrote:

FROM THE CAMP NEAR SAVANNAH,
February 10th, 1733.

To the Trustees for Establishing the Colony of Georgia in America:

GENTLEMEN: I gave you an account, in my last, of our arrival at Charleston. The Governor and Assembly have given us all possible encouragement. Our people arrived at Beaufort on the 20th of January, where I lodged them in some new barracks, built for the soldiers, while I went myself to view the Savannah river. I fixed upon a healthy situation, about ten miles from the sea. The river here forms a half moon, along the south side of which the banks are about forty foot high, and on the top flat, which they call a bluff. The plain high ground extends into the country five or six miles, and along the river side about a mile. Ships that draw twelve foot water can ride within ten yards of the bank. Upon the river side in the centre of this plain I have laid out the town. Opposite to it is an Island of very rich pasturage, which I think should be kept for the Trustee's cattle. The river is pretty wide, the water fresh, and from the Key of the town you see its whole course to the sea, with the Island of Tybee, which forms the mouth of the river; and the other way, you see the river for about six miles up into the country. The landscape is very agreeable, the stream being wide, and bordered with high woods on both sides. The whole people arrived here on the first of February. At night their tents were got up. Till the seventh we were taken up in unloading, and making a crane, which I then could not get finished, so took off the hands, and set some to the fortification, and began to fell the woods. I marked out the town and common; half of the former is already cleared, and the first house was begun yesterday in the afternoon. Not being able to get negroes, I have taken ten of the independent company to work for us, for which I make them an allowance. I send you a copy of the resolutions of the assembly, and the Governor and Council's letter to me. Mr. Whitaker has given us one hundred head of cattle. Colonel Bull, Mr. Barlow, Mr. St. Julian, and Mr. Woodward, are come up to assist us with some of their own servants. I am so taken up in looking after a hundred necessary things, that I write now short, but shall give you a more particular account hereafter. A little Indian nation, the only one within fifty miles, is not only at amity, but desires to be subjects of his Majesty, King George, to have lands given them among us, and to breed their children at our schools. Their Chief, and his beloved man, who is the second man in the nation, desire to be instructed in the Christian religion.

I am, gentlemen, your most obedient, humble servant,

JAMES OGLETHORPE.

He wrote, on the 12th:

Our people still lie in tents; there being only two clapboard houses built, and three sawed houses framed. Our crane, our battery of cannon, our magazine, are finished. This is all we have been able to do, by reason of the smallness of our number, of which many have been sick, and others unused to labour, though I thank God they are now pretty well, and we have not lost one since our arrival.

During this time the Governor, Council, and the people of South Carolina vied with one another in extending aid to the colonists, and in proof thereof we cite from the "MSS. account of benefactions made by South Carolina to the province of Georgia" the record of individual benefactions, the public ones having been already mentioned:

February—Colonel Bull came to Savannah with four laborers, and assisted the colony for a month, he himself measuring the scantling and setting out the work for the sawyers, and giving the proportion of the houses. Mr. Whitaker and his friends sent the colony one hundred head of cattle. Mr. St. Julian came to Savannah and staid a month, directing the people in building their houses and other work. Mr. Hume gave a silver boat and spoon for the first child born in Georgia, which being born of Mrs. Close, were given accordingly. Mr. Joseph Bryan, himself, with four of his sawyers, gave two months work in the colony. The inhabitants of Edisto sent sixteen sheep. Mr. Hammerton gave a drum. Mrs. Ann Drayton sent two pair of sawyers to work in the colony. Colonel Bull and Mr. Bryan came to Savannah with twenty servants, whose labor they gave to the colony. His Excellency Robert Johnson gave seven horses, valued at £25, Carolina currency.

Early in May, General Oglethorpe made a short trip to Charleston, S. C., where he met with a most cordial reception from the Governor and Legislature and from the people of that State. His solicitations for assistance were answered by the Assembly, which voted £10,000 currency, and the citizens of Charleston subscribed £1,000 currency, £500 of which were immediately paid down.

The General, well pleased with his hospitable reception and the liberal responses to his request for aid, returned to Savannah on the

21st of May, just in time to meet the representatives of the nine tribes of the Creek indians, who had assembled in solemn council to strengthen the provisional treaty which had been made with Tomichichi.

After the usual formalities, and a distribution of presents by Gen. Oglethorpe, Tomichichi addressed him as follows:

> Here is a little present; I give you a buffalo skin, adorned on the inside with the head and feathers of an eagle, which I desire you to accept, because the eagle is the emblem of speed and the buffalo of strength; the English are as swift as the bird and strong as the beast: since, like the former, they flew over vast seas to the uttermost parts of the earth; and like the latter, they are so strong that nothing can withstand them; the feathers of the eagle are soft, and signify love; the buffalo's skin is warm, and signifies protection; therefore, I hope the English will love and protect their little families.

A treaty was effected, providing that the indians should permit the Trustees to trade in their towns and that they should make restitution for any injuries done by the colonists to the indians, who, on their part, further agreed to allow the Trustees' people to make use of and possess all those lands which they had no occasion to use; not to molest nor rob any of the English, and, finally, "to keep the talk in their heads so long as the sun shall shine or the waters run into the rivers."

The ship James, Captain Yoakley, with several colonists on board, sailed up the Savannah and unloaded at the town a short time after the treaty. Captain Yoakley was given the prize which the Trustees had offered to the "first ship that should sail up the Savannah river and unload at the town."

By the seventh of July, one hundred and fifty more settlers arrived, a large number of whom came at their own expense; a large tract of land was cleared and a number of houses erected, and it was resolved to designate the town, wards, squares, and streets with formal ceremonies. Accordingly, on that day the emigrants assembled in front of Oglethorpe's tent, and after solemn religious ceremonies they proceeded to name the wards and assign the lots. Four wards were marked off and named: Heathcote, after Sir William Heathcote; Percival, after Lord Percival, the first President of the Trustees; Derby, after Earl of Derby; and Decker, after Sir William Decker. These wards were then divided into sixteen tithings, and named Digby, Carpenter, Frederick, Tyrconnel, More, Hucks, Tower, Heathcote, Eyles, Laroche, Vernon,

Beletha, Holland, Sloper, Wilmington, and Jekyll.* The five streets which intersected the wards and tithings at right angles were named in honor of the South Carolinians who aided the colony: Bull, Whitaker, Drayton, St. Julian, and Bryan. A square was also laid out, and as a mark of the respect and esteem which the colonists bore to Governor Johnson, of South Carolina, it was named after him. The assignment of the lots was next in order, which, after a display of considerable tact on the part of Oglethorpe to settle amicably the differences which arose in regard to the choice of locality, was accomplished by dinner-time. A bounteous repast was then partaken of.

After dinner, a town court of record was established, the bailiffs inducted into office, a jury empanneled, and the first court in Georgia held. This court was composed of three bailiffs, a recorder, acting as clerk, and twelve free-holders. The members of the court were ordered to wear, while sitting on the bench, majesterial gowns, those of the bailiff being purple, edged with fur, and that for the recorder being black, tufted. Messrs. Samuel Parker, Thomas Young, Joseph Cole, John Wright, John West, Timothy Bowling, John Milledge, Henry Close, Walter Fox, John Grady, James Carwell, and Richard Cannon composed the first grand jury.

Four days after these ceremonies a colony of Israelites arrived direct from London, named as follows: Dr. Nunis and his mother, Mrs. Nunis; Daniel Moses Nunis, Sipra Nunis, and Shem Noah, their servant; Mr. Henriques and wife, and Shem, their servant; Mr. and Mrs. Barnal; David Olivera; Jacob Olivera, wife, and three children, David, Isaac, and Leah; Aaron Depivea; Benjamin Gideon; Jacob Costa; David Depass and wife; Vene Real; Molena; David Moranda; Jacob Moranda; David Cohen, wife, and four children, Isaac, Hannah, Abigail, and Grace; Abraham Minis and wife, with their two daughters, Leah and Esther; Simeon Minis; Jacob Yowall; Benjamin Sheftall and wife; and Abraham DeLyon—all coming at their own expense.

Some persons in England became offended when the arrival of this party was reported, and wrote to the Trustees, stating that they would not contribute money for the support of the colony so long as the Hebrews remained. The Trustees wrote to the commis-

* Wilmington tithing was named after the Earl of Wilmington, and Jekyll after Sir Joseph Jekyll, Master of the Rolls.

sioners who had sent them over "to use their endeavors that the said Jews be removed from the colony of Georgia." Oglethorpe was also written to by the Trustees, who desired him "to use his endeavors to prevent their settling with any of the grantees." In reply, Oglethorpe praised their good conduct, and especially com-commended the skill and kindness of Dr. Nunis, who, since his arrival, had rendered valuable services to the sick colonists. Oglethorpe very wisely refused to move them, and time has proven that, had he complied with the request of the Trustees, the colony would have lost some of its most moral and industrious citizens. Although Oglethorpe did all he could to make their new-found home pleasant and comfortable, yet the civil disabilities under which they labored, the poor condition of the colony, and the advantages held out by the Charlestonians, induced all but three of the families, the Minises, DeLyons, and Sheftalls, to go to Charleston.

About this period the alligators, which had at first been frightened away by the bustle and noise made in building houses, felling trees, and the like, grew bold, and amused themselves by strolling about town at night, much to the annoyance and terror of the inhabitants. And "Mr. Oglethorpe," says the minutes of the Trustees, "to take off the terror which the people had for aligators, having wounded and caught one, twelve feet long, had him brought up to the town, and set the boys to beat him with sticks until he was beat to death."

From this time nothing of particular moment marked the history of Savannah until the 12th of March, 1734. On this day the Purysburgh arrived, bringing seventy-eight Salzburgers, who preferred to forsake their homes and seek new ones in a foreign and almost unknown land rather than give up their religion. Oglethorpe established them at a place twenty-four miles from Savannah, which they called Ebenezer.

After seeing the new colony settled, Oglethorpe left for England, carrying with him Tomichichi and one or two other indian chiefs, in order that they might become impressed with the strength and greatness of the English people, to strengthen the friendship of the indians, and also to interest the English in them. The colony was now left in charge of the bailiffs.

When Oglethorpe departed, there were, including the public buildings, ninety-one houses in the town, and the inhabitants were in a healthy and prosperous condition. The squares, streets, wards, and tithings laid out and named, the lots and houses assigned. A court-house, public mill and oven, a house for strangers, public store, parsonage-house, and guard-house built, a crane for hauling goods up the bluff erected, a fort and palisades to prevent an attack by land, and a battery on the bluff to prevent the approach of an enemy by water, established. A map of the town was drawn, by Peter Gordon, on the 29th of March, 1734, about a month previous to the General's departure, which gives an accurate description of the town as it then was. There was then no street between the river and the houses which were on the same line as those now located on the south side of Bay street. The places of note are marked on the map, and their sites can be readily pointed out at this time.

The four pine-trees under which the colonists pitched their four tents and slept the first night in Georgia were situated nearly on the edge of the bluff, between Bull and Whitaker streets, in front of where Robert Habersham & Co.'s commission house now stands.

The Stairs going up (1) were located a little east of the trees, about where Major P. H. Behn's commission house now stands.

Mr. Oglethorpe's Tent (2) was nearly under the cluster of trees.

The Crane and Bell (3), the first used to haul goods up the bluff and the other to call the colonists together for worship, work, and other purposes, were situated west of the trees, the crane on the edge of the bluff and the bell just in the rear of the crane; both on the site now occupied by the business house of L. J. Guilmartin & Co.

The Tabernacle and Court-house (4) was on Bull street, occupying the ground now occupied by the rear portion of the custom-house.

The Public Mill (5) was located on Bryan street, where now stands the establishment of U. Cranston.

The House for Strangers (6) stood on the site now occupied by the crockery and chinaware establishment of E. D. Smythe & Co., on the south side of St. Julian, second door east of Whitaker street.

The Public Oven (7) stood on the northeast corner of Congress and Whitaker streets, where now stands the extensive jewelry establishment of S. P. Hamilton.

The Draw-well (8) was situated in the centre of Bull street, where Congress Street lane intersects it.

The Lot for the Church (9) was laid out, but no church was built

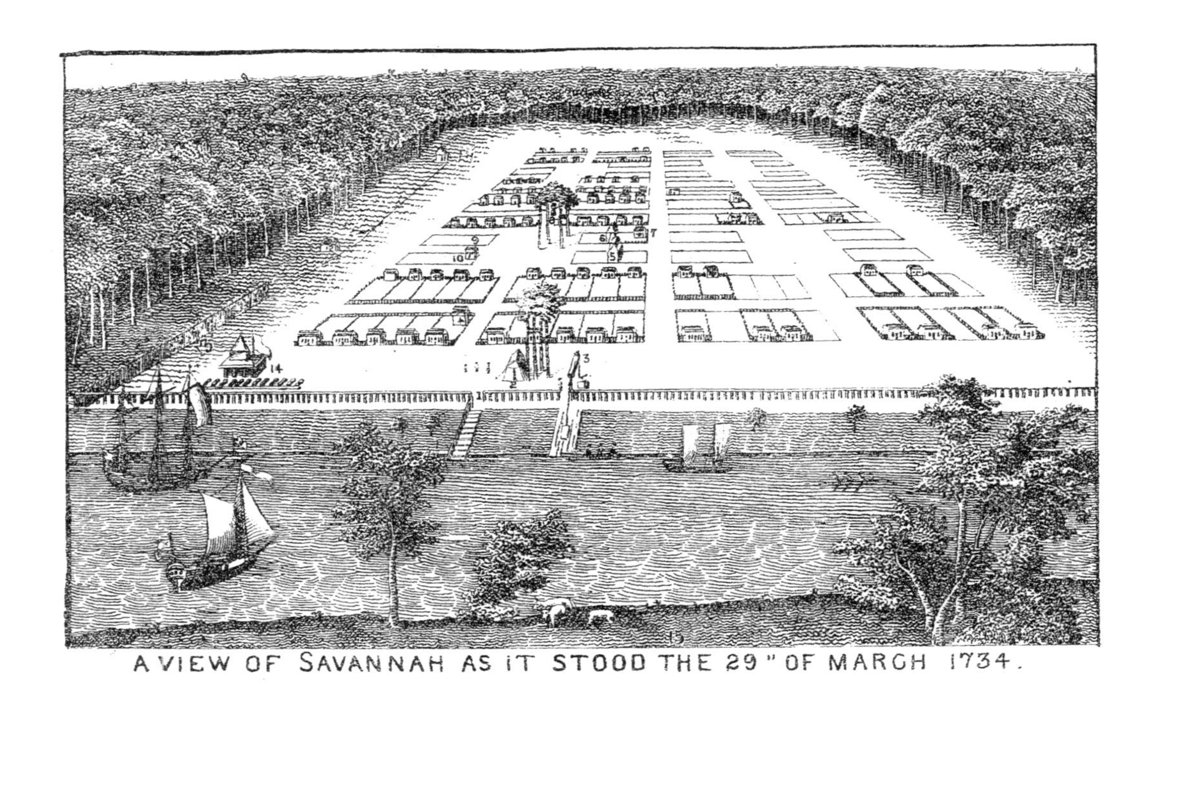

A VIEW OF SAVANNAH AS IT STOOD THE 29th OF MARCH 1734.

upon it for several years afterward. Christ church occupies the lot now.

The Public Store (10) was located where the State bank now stands.

The Fort (11) was situated on what is now the line of President street, and near Oglethorpe square.

The Parsonage-house (12) was situated in the middle of what is now Congress street, and on the west side of what is now Reynolds square.

The Palisades (13) were erected on a line extending from the bluff, at a point where now stands the business house of Hunter & Gammell, to the centre of what is now the block between Bay lane and Bryan street, and Drayton and Abercorn streets.

The Guard-house (14) and the battery of cannon were situated on the bluff, just at the foot of Drayton street.

Hutchinson's island (15) is seen on the opposite side of the river.

As has been stated, the colony was left under the charge of the three bailiffs, but one of them, John Causton, usurped all authority and made the other two simply his tools. His conduct was so overbearing that the colonists preferred charges against him, in which it was stated that he was of low origin and had become intoxicated with the powers vested in him, and was proud, haughty, and cruel; that he had threatened jurors whose verdicts did not correspond with his inclination or humor; that he had compelled eight freeholders, with an officer, to attend at the door of the court-house while it was in session, with their guns and bayonets, who had orders to rest their fire-locks as soon as he appeared; that he had threatened all, without distinction, who dared to oppose his arbitrary proceedings, or claimed their just rights and privileges, with the jail, stocks, and whipping-post, until he had rendered himself a terror to the people, and especially to jurors, who were afraid to act according to their consciences; that he had misapplied the public moneys; that everything had gone to ruin; "that the British nation was deceived (by him) with the fame of a happy, flourishing colony, and of its being free from that pest and scourge of mankind called lawyers, for the want of whose legal assistance the poor, miserable inhabitants are exposed to a more arbitrary government than ever was exercised in Turkey and Muscovy."

These representations of Causton's conduct caused his removal by the Trustees, and Mr. Gordon was sent over to assume the power and duties of chief magistrate. He possessed considerable ability and soon became a favorite with the people, and would have restored order and harmony, had not the cunning of old Causton pointed out an expedient to remove him. Causton was keeper of the public stores, and refused to allow Gordon either money or provisions. Gordon, having no way to support himself and family, was compelled to return to England six weeks after his arrival. His departure and the death of his successor, Mr. Durn, who died a few days after his appointment, left the field open for Causton to resume his arbitrary rule.

The impartiality of Judge Causton is shown in the trial of Captain Joseph Watson. Charges had been preferred against this militia officer by Causton, to the effect that he had stirred up animosities in the minds of the indians, and for this he was arraigned before the court, in which Causton was judge, witness, and advocate. The jury brought in a verdict that Watson was not guilty of any crime but that of having used some unguarded expressions. This verdict did not suit Causton, who ordered the jury to find another verdict, but they returned with the same; whereupon Causton again ordered them to retire and find the accused guilty and recommend him to the mercy of the court, imagining him to be a lunatic. The jury finally "found the accused guilty of lunacy;" whereupon Causton ordered him to prison, where he remained nearly three years without having sentence pronounced upon him.

During the absence of Oglethorpe attempts were made to cultivate grape vines and mulberry trees—to make wine and silk—in the "Trustees' garden," which had been laid out and enclosed at the east end of the town. The ground there was not adapted for the purpose, and those thus employed "found themselves cultivating a poor bit of sand which, in the heat of summer, would have roasted an egg." The trees did not flourish and the vines were parched with heat. The Trustees were notified of this, and another spot was selected. While the gardeners were so unsuccessful, Mr. Abram DeLyon, who had been a vigneron in Portugal, cultivated in his garden several varieties of grape, among which were the Oporto and Malaga, to great perfection.

The inhabitants of Savannah, in common with those of the other settlements, became discontented while Oglethorpe was absent, and upon his arrival in February, 1736, he experienced considerable difficulty in allaying the dissatisfaction.

Revs. John and Charles Wesley came over with Oglethorpe, and aided him in restoring harmony. On the Sunday after their arrival, Rev. John Wesley* (afterward the founder of Methodism) preached his first sermon in America, his text being from the Epistle of the day—13th chapter 1st Corinthians—and christian charity his theme.

* The popularity of this divine was very great with the people of Savannah. On one occasion during his stay in the colony a ball and public prayers were announced to take place at the same time. "At the hour appointed," says a chronicler of the times, "the church was full, while the ball-room was so empty that the entertainment could not go forward."

CAPTER II.

Savannah in 1736 — Its Situation — Houses and People — Laws and Customs — Town Lots and Squares — Public Buildings — Arrival of Rev. George Whitfield and Mr. James Habersham — Burial of Tomichichi — Judge Causton again Introduced — The Inhabitants Puzzled — Building of the Orphan House — Condition of Savannah in 1743 — Establishment of the First Commercial and Manufacturing Houses — Hostile Indians in Savannah — Organization of the Union Society — Meeting of the First General Assembly of Georgia — First General Muster.

Mr. Francis Moore visited the colony in 1736, and wrote an account* of his visit, in which he described Savannah as follows:

Savannah is about a mile and a quarter in circumference; it stands upon the flat of a hill; the bank of the river (which they in barbarous English call a bluff) is steep and about forty-five feet perpendicular, so that all heavy goods are brought up by a crane, an inconvenience designed to be remedied by a bridge-wharf, and an easy ascent, which, in laying out the town, care was taken to allow room for, there being a very wide strand between the first row of houses and the river. From this strand there is a very pleasant prospect; you can see the river wash the foot of the hill, which is a hard, clear, sandy beach a mile in length; the water is fresh, and the river one thousand foot wide. Eastward you see the river increased by the northern branch which runs around Hutchinson's island, and the Carolina shore beyond it, and the woody islands at the sea, which closes the prospect at ten or twelve miles distance. Over against it is Hutchinson's island, great part of which is open ground, where they mow hay for the Trustees' horses and cattle. The rest is woods, in which there are many bay trees eighty foot high. Westward you see the river winding between the woods, with little islands in it, for many miles.

The town of Savannah is built of wood; all the houses of the first forty freeholders are of the same size with that Mr. Oglethorpe lives in,† but there are great numbers built since—I believe one hundred or one hundred and fifty; many of these are much larger; some of two or three stories high, the boards plained and painted. The houses stand on large lots, sixty foot in front by ninety foot in depth; each lot has a fore and back street to it; the lots are fenced in with split poles; some people have palisades of split wood before their doors, but the generality have been wise enough not to throw away their money, which in this country, laid out in husbandry, is capable of great improvements.

There are several people of good substance in the town, who came at

---

* The account is published in the "Collections of the Georgia Historical Society."

† Sixteen by twenty-four feet.

their own expense, and also several of those who came over on the Charity are in a very thriving way; but this is observed, that the most substantial people are the most frugal, and make the least show, and live at the least expense. There are some also who have made but little or bad use of the benefits they received, idling away their times, whilst they had their provisions from the public store, or else working for hire, earning from two shillings, the price for a laborer, to four or five shillings, the price of a carpenter, per diem, and spending that money in rum and good living, thereby neglecting to improve their lands, so that when their time of receiving their provisions from the public ceased they were in no forwardness to maintain themselves out of their own lands. As they chose to be hirelings when they might have improved for themselves, the consequence of that folly forces them now to work for their daily bread. These are generally discontented with the country; and if they have run themselves in debt, their creditors will not let them go away till they have paid. Considering the number of people, there are but few of these. The industrious ones have throve beyond expectation; most of them that have been there three years, and many others, have houses in the town, which those that let have for the worst ten pounds per annum, and the best for thirty pounds. Those who have cleared their five-acre lots have made a very great profit out of them by greens, roots, and corn. Several have improyed the cattle they had at first, and have now five or six tame cows; others who, to save the trouble of feeding them, let them go into the woods can rarely find them, and when they are brought up, one of them will not give half the quantity of milk which another cow fed near home will give. Their houses are built at a pretty large distance from one another, for fear of fire; the streets are very wide, and there are great squares left at proper distances for markets and other conveniences. Near the river side is a guard-house inclosed with palisades a foot thick, where there are nineteen or twenty cannons mounted and a continual guard kept by the freeholders.

The town is governed by three bailiffs, and has a recorder, register, and a town court, which is holden every six weeks, where all matters, civil and criminal, are decided by grand and petit juries, as in England; but there are no lawyers allowed to plead for him; nor no attorneys to take money, but (as in old times in England) every man pleads his own cause. In case it should be an orphan, or one that can not speak for themselves, there are persons of the best substance in the town appointed by the Trustees to take care of the orphans and to defend the helpless, and that without fee or reward, it being a service that each that is capable must perform in his turn.

They have some laws and customs that are peculiar to Georgia; one is that all brandies and distilled liquors are prohibited under severe penalties; another is; that no slavery is allowed, nor negroes; a third, that all persons who go among the indians must give security for their good behavior; because the indians, if any injury is done to them and they can not kill the man that does it, expect satisfaction from the government, which if not procured they break out into war by killing the first white man they conveniently can.* No victualler or alehouse-keeper can give any credit, so

* All west of Jefferson street from the bluff to the south side of South

consequently can not recover any debt. The freeholds have all been entailed, which has been very fortunate for the place. If people could have sold, the greatest part, before they knew the value of their lots, would have parted with them for a trifling condition, and there were not wanting rich men who employed agents to monopolize the whole town.

In order to maintain many people, it was proper that the land should be divided into small portions, and to prevent the uniting them by marriage or purchase. For every time two lots were united the town loses a family, and the inconveniency of this shows itself at Savannah, notwithstanding the care of the Trustees to prevent it. They suffered the moity of the lots to descend to the widows during their lives; those who remarried to men who had lots of their own, by uniting two lots made one be neglected; for the strength of hands who could take care of one was not sufficient to look to and improve two. These uncleared lots are a nuisance to their neighbors. The trees which grow upon them shade the lots, the beasts take shelter in them, and for want of clearing the brooks which pass through them the lands above are often prejudiced by floods. To prevent all these inconveniences, the first regulation of the Trustees was a strict Agrarian law, by which all the lands near towns should be divided, 50 acres to each freeholder. The quantity of land by experience seems rather too much, since it is impossible that one poor family can tend so much land. If this allotment is too much, how much more inconvenient would the uniting of two be? To prevent it the Trustees grant the land in tail-male, that on the expiring of a male line they may regrant it to such man, having no other lot, as shall be married to the next female heir of the deceased as is of good character. This manner of dividing prevents, also, the sale of lands, and the rich thereby monopolizing the country.

Each freeholder has a lot in town sixty foot by ninety foot, besides which he has a lot beyond the common of five acres for a garden. Every ten houses make a tithing, and to every tithing there is a mile square, which is divided into twelve lots, besides roads; each freeholder of the tithing has a lot or farm of forty-five acres there and two lots† are reserved by the Trustees in order to defray the charge of the public. The town is laid out for two hundred and forty freeholds; the quantity of land necessary for that number is twenty-four square miles; every forty houses in town make a ward, to which four square miles in the country belong; each ward has a constable, and under him four tithing-men.

Where the town land ends the villages begin; four villages make a ward out, which depends upon one of the wards within the town. The use of this is, in case a war should happen, the villages without may have places in the town to bring their cattles and families into for refuge, and for that purpose there is a square left in every ward big enough for the outwards to encamp in. There is a ground also kept around about the town ungranted, in order for the fortifications whenever occasion shall require. Beyond the villages

---

Broad street, thence to the eastern limits of the city, was the boundary. On the trees at intervals along this boundary line, planks, one side painted white the other red, were nailed to "show the people they could not go over that mark to cut wood, as it belonged to the indians."

† These lots were called "Trust Lots."

commences lots of five hundred acres; these are granted upon terms of keeping the servants, &c. There is near the town to the east a garden belonging to the Trustees consisting of ten acres; the situation is delightful, one half of it upon the top of the hill, the foot of which the Savannah river washes, and from it you see the woody islands in the sea. The remainder of the garden is the side and some plain low ground at the foot of the hill, where several fine springs broke out.

The constant arrival of persons from England and other places, to settle in the various settlements in Georgia, contributed to swell the population of Savannah, many being so well pleased with the town that they refused to go further, and made it their home. Consequently, in 1738, we find that the town has been considerably enlarged, new streets, wards, and squares laid out and new houses built. Notwithstanding this manifest improvement in the population and dimensions in the town, very little if any attention was paid to the public buildings, as will be seen from the following account of them written at that time:

The public works in this town are: 1. A Court-house, being one handsome room, with a piache on three sides. This likewise serves as a church for divine service, none having been ever built, notwithstanding the Trustees in their public acts acknowledged the receipt of about seven hundred pounds sterling from charitable persons for that express purpose.

2. Opposite the Court-house stands the log house or prison (which is the only one remaining of five or six that have been successively built in Savannah), that place of terror and support of absolute power in Georgia.

3. Nigh thereto is a house built of logs, at a very great charge, as was said, for the Trustees' steward; the foundation below ground is rotten, as the whole fabric must be in a short time, for the roof being flat the rain comes in at all parts of it.

4. The Storehouse, which has been many times altered and amended at a very great charge, and it now serves as a store for the private benefit of one or two.

5. The Guard-house, which was first built on the bluff, soon decayed, as did a second, through improper management, this now standing being the third. Several flag-staffs were likewise erected, the last of which, according to common report, cost £50 sterling.

6. A Public Mill for grinding corn was first erected, at a considerable expense, in one square of the town, but in about three years time (without doing the least service) it fell to the ground. In another square of the town a second was set up, at a far greater expense, but never finished, and is now erased and converted into a house for entertaining the indians and other such like uses.

7. Several of the houses which were built by freeholders, for want of heirs male, are fallen to the Trustees (even to the prejudice of the lawful creditors of the deceased) and are disposed of as the General thinks proper.

At least two hundred lots were taken up in Savannah, about one hundred and seventy of which were built upon.

Rev. George Whitfield, who had secured from the Trustees a tract of land near Savannah for the purpose of building an asylum for the poor children, arrived in May, 1737, accompanied by Mr. James Habersham.

In October of this year a grand council of the chiefs of the four towns of the Creek nation was held in Savannah, and with the assistance of Tomichichi another treaty was arranged, by which the indians agreed to form a friendly alliance with the English and assist them against their enemies. This was the last opportunity that Tomichichi had to show his friendship to the colonists, who were indebted greatly to him for protection. He died the following October. In compliance with his request that he might be buried among the English, his remains were brought from his place above the town in a canoe, and were met at the bluff by Oglethorpe, the the civil authorities, and the citizens, all of whom, out of respect, assembled to assist in the funeral obsequies. A procession was formed, and the corpse, with Oglethorpe and Colonel Stephens, the President, as pall-bearers, was escorted to Percival * square, minute guns being fired from the Battery the while. As the body was lowered into the earth three volleys of musketry were fired by the militia.

The close of 1739 introduces John Causton again; he had continued his arbitrary measures up to this time. William Stephens, Thomas Christie, and Thomas Jones, Esqs., were appointed to examine his accounts, which were never satisfactorily settled, and Causton was removed for mal-practice in office. This duty was hardly over before the services of Mr. Stephens were again called for.

The Council of the Trustees had met in London and adopted a series of long resolutions relating to the grants and tenure of lands in Georgia, which were incomprehensible. They were published in the Charleston papers, but as they were not understood Stephens was requested to read and explain them as he went along. This he proceeded to do one day at the court-house, but, though he exerted his utmost abilities, failed to explain them satisfactorily. After he gave up, one of the settlers ludicrously remarked that "the

* Now Court-house square.

whole paper consisted of *males* and *tails*,* and that all the lawyers in London would not be able to bring the meaning down to his comprehension, and that he understood as little of its meaning then as he had when Stephens began"—others wished to "know how often these two words had occurred in the resolutions; that the number ought to be preserved as a curiosity; and that the author of the resolutions ought to be lodged in bedlam for lunacy."

The building of the "Orphan House" was commenced in 1740, and located on what was then described to be a sandy bluff, near the sea-shore, and was named Bethesda. The house was constructed under the superintendence of Mr. Joseph Habersham, who took a warm interest in the laudable undertaking. An account of this "noble charity" will be found under the head of "Bethesda."

The invasion of Georgia by the Spaniards from Florida occurred at this period, and caused many people to leave Savannah, fearing that the enemy would reach it and massacre the inhabitants. Owing to the generalship of Oglethorpe and the bravery of the colonists, who volunteered to defend their homes, the enemy were repulsed before arriving within many miles. This war retarded the settlers from making any improvements, and at its close Savannah was in anything but a flourishing condition, yet under the smiling influences of peace the settlers again went to work and soon placed the town upon a better footing than ever before. When Oglethorpe finally left the colony, in 1743, there were three hundred and fifty-three houses, exclusive of the public buildings. Among these were a number of elegant houses surrounded by large gardens.

Mr. James Habersham, of whom we have before had occasion to speak, together with Mr. Charles Harris, established here, in 1744, the first commercial house in Georgia. The firm was known as Harris & Habersham,† and gave great encouragement to the planters, from whom they purchased lumber, hogs, poultry, deer skins, &c., a cargo of which, valued at $10,000, was shipped to England in 1749. This was the first attempt to commence a foreign trade. A letter written by Mr. Habersham to a friend in England, expressing his views upon the advantages of agriculture and commerce to the colony, fell into the hands of the Trustees, and they were led by it to think seriously upon the subject and to adopt

* In-tail-male.

† Their place of business was close to the water's edge, and just in rear of where Robert Habersham & Co.'s commission house now stands.

measures which tended to advance those interests. Previous to this the colonists had become weary of attempting to produce silk and wine, for which purpose the colony had been established, and neglected the gardens where the vines and mulberry trees had been planted; and many of them petitioned the Trustees to abandon the idea of producing silk and wine exclusively and appropriate money for the purposes of agriculture and commerce. Notwithstanding the experience of fourteen years had shown the Trustees that their favorite projects had come to nothing, they refused to grant the requests in the petition, and paid no attention to the subjects mentioned, until they came into the possession of Mr. Habersham's letter.*

Even then they did not altogether abandon the cherished hope that Georgia was a "silk and wine growing colony," for they made another effort, in 1750, to encourage the growth of silk, offering large bounties to all who would engage in it; and in the year following a filature, or house for the manufacture of silk, was built on the west side of Reynold's square, on the ground now occupied by "Cassell's Row."

In our efforts to give the reader an accurate account of the establishment of the first commercial and manufacturing houses in Savannah, and of the first exports from it, we passed over an occurrence which we venture to assert was never forgotten by those of the inhabitants who witnessed it, as for a time they were completely at the mercy of the indians, who, thirsting for the lands occupied by the whites, assembled in Savannah and demanded a relinquishment of them.

It will be remembered that through the influence of the half-breed woman, Mary Musgrove, Oglethorpe obtained permission from the indians to settle upon Yamacraw bluff. After the death of John Musgrove, which occurred three years after the landing of Oglethorpe, Mary married a Captain Mathews, who died in 1742. Shortly after his death Mary married again, Rev. Thomas Bosomworth, a clergyman of the Church of England, at the time in the employ of the "Society for the Propagation of Christian Knowledge," being the happy man. Previous to this alliance Mary had been upon the most friendly terms with the colonists.

* So well pleased were the Trustees with the arguments used in this letter, that they immediately appointed the author a member of the Council in Georgia.

Her conduct was now entirely the reverse. Before she stood as a mediatrix between the whites and indians; now she did all in her power to excite dissension between them. This change was due to Bosomworth. He laid claims to the islands of Ossaba, Sapelo, and St. Catherine, and for a few trifles obtained them from Malatchee, the brother of Mary, and who, because of his fickle temper, was by the indians compared to the wind. Bosomworth had previously gone through the farce of crowning Malatchee king, and about fifteen other chiefs "head warriors and beloved men" of seven different towns, all of whom, on the 14th of December, 1747, signed a paper acknowledging Malatchee the right and lawful prince, and pledging themselves to "ratify and confirm every act and deed of his." Bosomworth, by his unthriftiness, soon became entangled in debt, and to extricate himself, encouraged his wife to assume the title of an independent empress, which she did and summoned a meeting of the Creeks, before whom, in a violent harrangue, she insisted upon the justice of her pretensions. The indians were aroused to a high pitch of excitement by this speech, and pledged themselves "to stand by her to their last drop of blood." This object being accomplished, Bosomworth became bold and insolent, and in 1749 he and Mary, with a large body of savages in their train, marched toward Savannah, he having previously sent a messenger to Colonel William Stephens, President of the Council, to inform him "that Mary had assumed her right of sovereignty over the whole territories of the Upper and Lower Creeks, and to demand that all lands belonging to them be instantly relinquished, for as she was the hereditary and rightful Queen of both nations and could command every man of them to follow her, in case of refusal she had determined to extirpate the settlement."

These bold pretentions and threats alarmed the President and Council, but they determined to put the town in the best posture of defence possible, and summoned the militia to place themselves under arms, which was done, but the whole force amounted to only one hundred and seventy men. A messenger was sent to Mary, while several miles distant from town, to ascertain whether she was serious in such wild pretensions, and if possible to make her dismiss her followers and abandon her design. Mary was inflexible and resolute, and the President resolved to receive them with firmness. As the indians entered the town, on the 10th of August,

1749, the militia met them, and Captain Noble Jones, commanding a troop of horse, halted them and demanded whether they came with hostile or friendly intent; to which the indians made no satisfactory reply, whereupon he told them that they must leave their arms there, as he had orders not to permit an armed man of them to set his foot within the town. Some further parley ensued, which resulted in the indians reluctantly grounding their arms. The indians then marched in town to the Parade, Bosomworth in his canonical robes, with his queen by his side, heading the procession.

Arriving at the Parade, the militia saluted them by firing fifteen rounds from cannon and with volleys of musketry. The President then demanded their intentions in visiting the town in so large a body when they had not been sent for by any person in lawful authority. The warriors, in reply, said that they had heard it was the intention of the English to seize Mary and send her captive over the great water; that they intended no harm, and begged that their arms might be restored to them; and then, after consulting with Bosomworth and his wife, they would return and settle all public affairs. Their muskets were returned, but no ammunition was given them.

The Council was then dismissed, to reassemble on the following day. In terror and alarm the inhabitants passed the night, only to be more alarmed when morning came, for then the indians, who had been aroused by the private harangues of the queen and Bosomworth during the night, became very surly and ran in a tumultuous manner up and down the streets, seemingly bent upon mischief. The confusion became very great. The militia were under arms, and therefore away from the houses. The women and children, fearing that if they remained at home they would be butchered, crowded into the streets, thereby increasing the confusion; during which a false rumor was circulated that the indians had cut off President Stephens' head with a tomahawk. The inhabitants became so exasperated at this that it was with great difficulty the officers prevented them from firing upon the savages. Bosomworth was immediately seized and confined, which made Mary frantic. She threatened vengeance against the magistrates and the colony, and ordered every white man to depart from her territories. She cursed Oglethorpe and asserted that his treaties were fraudulent, and, stamping her foot violently upon the ground, swore by her Maker that the whole earth on which she trode was her own.

Observing that no peaceable arrangement could be made with the indians while under the eye of their pretended queen, President Stephens had her privately arrested and confined with her husband. The chief promoters of the conspiracy being out of the way, negotiations were entered into with the indians. A bounteous feast was prepared, and while the warriors were thus entertained they were informed of the wicked designs of Bosomworth and his wife: "that the former was involved in debt and wanted not only their lands but also a large share of the royal bounty to satisfy his creditors, most of whom lived in Carolina; that the king's presents were intended only for the indians, on account of their useful services and firm attachment to him during former wars; that the lands adjoining the town were reserved for them to encamp upon when they came to visit their beloved friends in Savannah, and the three maritime islands to hunt upon when they should come to bathe in the salt waters; that neither Mary nor her husband had any right to those lands which were the common property of the Creek nations; that the great king had ordered the President to defend their right to them, and expected that all his subjects, both white and red, would live together like brethren."

This speech and the kindness of the people had the desired effect, even Malatchee with the other chieftains being convinced; but in a few hours afterward he, having in the meantime had a talk with Bosomworth and Mary, was seduced and drawn over again to support their chimerical claims, and while the President was distributing the royal presents, which were intended to further conciliate the indians, Malatchee arose and in a violent and excited tone protested that Mary possessed the country before General Oglethorpe, and all the lands belonged to her as queen and head of the Creeks; that it was only by her permission the English were allowed to settle on them; that her word was the voice of the whole nation, consisting of about three thousand warriors, and every one would take up the hatchet in defence of her right. He then handed a paper to the President which had evidently been written by Bosomworth. It was substantially the same as the speech made by Malatchee, and discovered in the plainest manner the ambitious views and wicked intrigues of Bosomworth. The whole Board was struck with astonishment when the letter was read, and Malatchee, observing their uneasiness, begged that it might be returned to him, as he did not know it was bad talk, and promised to return it to the person who had given it to him.

It was necessary to remove the impression made by Malatchee's speech, and the indians were assembled; the President then addressed them, stating the benefits the indians and whites had mutually derived from each other, and showing that it would be to their interest to remain in peace and harmony, and not to allow the wicked Bosomworth to interrupt the fraternal relations which then existed. The President was not allowed to finish his speech, for the indians desired him to stop, stating that their eyes were opened, and though Bosomworth desired to break the chain of friendship they were determined to hold it fast, and begged that all might smoke the pipe of peace. This was done, rum drank, and presents distributed.

The general joyousness which followed induced the President and Council to believe that all differences were amicably settled, and were rejoicing in the restoration of their former friendly inter. course with the Creeks, when Mary, drunk and disappointed in her views, furiously rushed in the midst of the assemblage and told the President he had nothing to do with the indians, and would be convinced of it to his cost. The President ordered her to cease her remarks; that if she did not he would again imprison her. This infuriated her, and turning to Malatchee she told him what had been said. Malatchee immediately seized his arms, and calling upon the rest to follow his example, dared any man to touch the queen. In a moment the whole house was a scene of uproar and tumult and all the whites present expected nothing but instant death. Captain Jones, who commanded the guard, immediately interposed and ordered the indians to deliver up their arms, which they reluctantly did. Mary was then conveyed to a private room. A guard was placed over her and all further intercourse with the savages denied her during their stay in Savannah.

The husband was sent for, in order that he might be reasoned with and convinced of the folly of his pretensions and the dangerous consequences which might arise if he persisted in them. So soon as he made his appearance before the President and Council he commenced a tirade of abuse against them, and despite the kindness shown him and the arguments used to persuade him into submission, he remained obstinate and contumacious, and protested he would stand forth in vindication of his wife's right to the last extremity, and that Georgia should soon feel the weight of her vengeance.

The indians were persuaded to leave town after both of their leaders were confined, thus happily relieving the inhabitants, who were wearied out with constant watching and harassed with frequent alarms. Shortly after their departure Bosomworth and Mary repented of their folly and asked the pardon of the Magistrates and the people. Thus ended, without bloodshed, one of the most formidable demonstrations ever made by the indians in Georgia. This happy result of the difficulty was only obtained by the exercise of the greatest prudence and bravery, without which the people of Savannah would have fallen a sacrifice to the indiscriminate vengeance of the savages.* Bosomworth was afterward given the island of St. Catherine, upon which he and Mary lived for several years.

In 1750 the Union Society, of which further mention will hereafter be made, was founded by Richard Milledge, an Episcopalian, Peter Tondee, a Catholic, and Benjamin Sheftall, an Israelite; hence the name "Union Society."

The first General Assembly of Georgia met in Savannah on the 15th of January, 1751, sixteen representatives present. Francis Harris, John Milledge, William Francis, and William Russell were from the Savannah district. Francis Harris was chosen speaker. A number of complaints were made by the Assembly (which seems to have had no more power than a grand jury of our day) to the Council, of which Henry Parker was President and James Habersham Secretary. The complaints were:

1st. The want of a proper pilot boat.

2d. The want of leave to erect a building under the bluff for the convenience of boat-crews, negroes, etc.

3d. The want of standard weights, scales, and measures.

4th. The want of a survey of the river.

5th. The want of an order to prevent masters of vessels from heaving ballast, etc., into the river.

6th. The want of a commissioner for regulating pilots and pilotage.

7th. The want of an inspector and sworn packer to inspect the produce of the colony.

8th. The want of a clerk of the market.

9th. The want of regulations for the guard.

10th. The want of proper officers to command the militia.

11th. The want of repairs to the court-house.

---

* The account of this demonstration was condensed from a work published in London, in 1779, by Dr. Hewitt.

The Council replied that the first should be represented to the Trustees; to the second, a place shall be laid out; to the third, applied for by the Board and may be expected; to the fourth, to be done as soon as a proper person can be found; to the fifth, an order to be published; to the sixth, seventh, eighth, and tenth, to be appointed; to the ninth, to be remedied; eleventh, to be immediately done.

After the adjournment of the Assembly the Council, in pursuance of its promise to that body to organize the militia, issued an order for all who possessed three hundred acres and upward of land to appear well accoutred on horseback as cavalry; and those who owned less property armed as foot. The first general muster took place in Savannah on the 13th of June, 1751. There were about two hundred and twenty horse and foot, well armed and equipped; and, says a colonial record, "they behaved well and made a pretty appearance."

CHAPTER III.

Arrival of Governor Reynolds — His Opinion of the Town — Burning of the Filature — Arrival of Governor Ellis — A Deadly Blow Aimed at Savannah's Commercial Prospects — Another Treaty with the Indians — Construction of the First Wharf — Arrival of Governor Wright and Departure of Governor Ellis — Establishment of the First Newspaper and Post-office — The Stamp Act Excitement — Arrival of the Stamps — The Liberty Boys Threaten to Destroy them — The Governor Frightened — He is Burnt in Effigy — Savannah in 1765 — South Carolinians Destroy Vessels Bound to Savannah — Savannah Merchants Refuse to Import Goods from England — Increase of the Spirit of Rebellion — Seizure of the King's Magazine — Raising of the First Liberty Pole — Liberal Views of the Citizens.

On the 29th of October, 1754, there were public and joyous demonstrations of every character in Savannah, caused by the arrival of Governor John Reynolds, who had been appointed Governor of the colony by the English government, to which the Trustees had resigned their charter in 1752. The arrival of the new Governor was totally unexpected. But as he ascended the bluff he was received with every manifestation of joy. At night there were bonfires and illuminations. The following day he was duly installed into office, and his commission as Captain-General and Vice-Admiral of the province was read to the militia, who were under arms before the council chamber.* The militia listened with profound attention, and afterward fired several rounds of musketry. A public dinner was then given, at which the new Governor was entertained by the council and principal inhabitants.

The Governor had formed an exaggerated opinion of the state of the colony, especially of its metropolis, but was soon undeceived, as is shown by his first letter to the Board of Trade in London, in which he spoke of Savannah as follows:

Savannah is well situated, and contains about one hundred and fifty houses, all wooden ones, very small and mostly old. The biggest was used for the

---

* The council chamber was situated on the lot where now stands the residence of Captain T. F. Screven, fronting on Reynolds square.

meeting of the president and assistants, and where I sat in council for a few days, but one end fell down whilst we were all there, and obliged us to move to a kind of shed, behind the court-house, which being quite unfit, I have given orders, with the advice of the council, to fit up the shell of a house, which was lately built for laying up the silk but was never made use of, being very ill-calculated for that purpose, but it will make a tolerably good house for the Assembly to meet in and for a few offices besides. The prison, being only a small wooden house, without security, I have also ordered to be mended and some locks and bolts to be put on for the present.

In 1757 one thousand and fifty pounds of raw silk were received at the filature in Savannah. The following year the filature was burnt. Its contents, a large quantity of silk and seven thousand and forty pounds of cocoons, or silk-balls, were consumed.*.

In February of 1757 Henry Ellis, who had been appointed Governor of the province, arrived in Savannah. He was appointed as successor to Governor Reynolds, who had been completely ruled by his secretary, William Little. Little made himself very obnoxious to the people, and amid the bonfires, illuminations, and other demonstrations of joy which marked Governor Ellis' arrival, he was burnt in effigy "as a tyrant in himself and a promoter of it in his master." A prominent feature of the occasion was the drill of a company of thirty juvenile soldiers, under command of their schoolmaster. They presented to the Governor the following address:

SIR—The youngest militia of this province presume, by their captain, to salute your Honor on your arrival. Although we are of too tender years to comprehend the blessing a good Governor is to a province, our parents will doubtless experience it in its utmost extent, and their grateful tale shall fix your name dear in our memories.

The warm reception and hospitable treatment of the Governor by the people of Savannah was not reciprocated by him. He aimed a deadly blow at her prospects as a commercial town, by endeavoring to have the capital of the colony removed to Hardwicke,† claiming that it possessed decided advantages over Savannah because of the depth of water there, its more central position, and its greater distance from Charleston; the proximity of which, he urged, restricted the commerce of Savannah. Fortunately for Sa-

---

* The filature was rebuilt and used for the manufacture of silk several years. It was afterward used as a city hall and a public house. It was destroyed by fire in 1839.

† Hardwicke was situated near the mouth of the Ogeechee river in Bryan county.

vannah, his project, which had been suggested by his predecessor, was not carried into effect, but the agitation of the proposed plan injured the town; the inhabitants, thinking that it was shortly to be deserted, neglected to enlarge and beautify it; the public buildings were not repaired; the filature was in a "tumble-down condition;" the church was so decayed that it would have fallen but for the support rendered by props; and the prison "was shocking to humanity."

The 25th of October, 1757, was another day of note in the history of Savannah. Then a council was held in the town with a large body of chiefs and head men of the Upper and Lower Creek nations for the purpose of defeating the objects of the French, who were intriguing with the indians and exciting them to hostility against the English, whose military force was quadrupled by that of the indians. The Governor intended to impress the indians with ideas of the strength of the English, and previous to their arrival had the guns in all of the batteries about the towns loaded and flags unfurled over them. The regiment of militia, Colonel Noble Jones commanding, was paraded under arms in town. Captain John Milledge, with a company of rangers, met the indians and acted as an escort for them. When near the town, they were met by Captain Bryan and a large number of citizens, who welcomed them and supplied them with needed refreshment; after which, the inhabitants and guests marched into town, the citizens on horseback in front. At the forts a salute of thirteen guns were fired. Here the citizens paused and allowed the indians to pass by. They were then received by Colonel Jones at the head of the foot-militia. With drums beating and colors flying, the cavalcade proceeded to the council chamber, passing by the Governor's house, where a salute was fired by a battery placed in front, which was followed by the guns in the water-battery and on the ships in the river. At the council chamber another salute was fired by the Virginia Blues. The Governor met them here, and with hands extended said:

MY FRIENDS AND BROTHERS—Behold my hands and arms. Our common enemies, the French, have told you they are red to the elbows. View them; do they speak the truth? Let your own eyes witness. You see they are white, and could you see my heart you would find it as pure, but very warm and true to you, my friends. The French tell you, whoever shakes my hands will immediately be struck with disease and die. If you believe this lying, foolish talk, do n't touch me. If you do not, I am ready to embrace you.

The indians, before the last words of this most appropriate speech were uttered, rushed forward, and shaking the Governor's hands, declared that they had often been deceived by the French, but would not be so again. Other speeches of a friendly character followed, and the council resulted in establishing the utmost harmony and confidence between the two races.

Up to this period, twenty-six years after the settlement of Savannah, there was no wharf built. The few vessels that came here sailed as close to land as the depth of water would permit and threw the lighter articles on the bank, landing the heavier ones in small boats. Feeling the necessity of having a wharf, the subject was discussed, and this year one was constructed by Thomas Eaton, under the direction of John G. William DeBrahm, the Surveyor-General of the southern provinces of North America. The builder was advised, which advice he followed, "to drive two rows of piles as far asunder as he desired his wharf to be wide, and as far toward the river as low-water mark; secure their tops with plates and to trunnel planks within on the piles. This done, then to brace the insides with dry walls of stones intermingled with willow twigs. In the same manner to shut up the ends of the two rows with a like front along the stream, to build inside what cellars he had occasion for, then to fill up the remainder with the sand nearest at hand, out of the bluff or high shore of the stream under the bay." This wharf, tradition asserts, was constructed on the river a little west of the steps by which the inhabitants went up and down the bluff—most probably about midway between Bull and Whitaker streets. The plan by which it was constructed was followed several years. The construction of this wharf appears to have benefitted the town, for during the following year forty-one vessels were entered—many more than ever before; and during the year 1766, six years after, one hundred and seventy-one were entered.

Governor Ellis, by his own request, was removed from office, and was succeeded by Sir James Wright, who arrived in Savannah in October, 1760, when he was received with the usual formalities. There were not many manifestations of joy, because of the general distress which prevailed owing to the departure of Governor Ellis, who, by his kind and just administration, had endeared himself not only to the inhabitants of Savannah but to the whole colony. The Union Society presented him an address and a handsome piece of plate "as a token of the public gratitude of the inhabitants of Savannah."

On the 20th of March, 1761, King George III issued an order conferring upon Governor Wright full executive powers, with the title of Captain-General and Governor-in-Chief, but such was the slow transit between the two countries that it did not reach him until the 28th of January, 1762, nearly a year after its issue, on which day it was promulgated and made the occasion of a general holiday. Colonel Noble Jones' regiment of militia was drawn up in Johnson square, and after hearing the order read fired a salute, which was answered by the fort and the ships in the river. At night the Governor gave a ball to the ladies, at which, says a chronicler of the time, "there was the most numerous and brilliant appearance ever known in the town." Altogether, it was a brilliant affair, and "there never was an occasion on which the joy and satisfaction of the people were more apparent."

A printing press, the first in Georgia, was established here early in 1763, and on the seventh of April the "Georgia Gazette" paper was issued; the following year a post-office was also established, and Robert Bolton, Esq., appointed postmaster.

The obnoxious Stamp act, which received the Royal assent in 1765, excited all of the colonies to a spirit of resistance, and in response to a circular addressed by the Assembly of Massachusetts, showing the importance of union among the aggrieved colonies and soliciting the formation of a general congress, to meet in New York, Alexander Wylly, speaker of the Commons House of Assembly, convened the Assembly here on the second of September, 1765. This body, in reply to the circular, stated that their hearty co-operation in all measures for the support of the rights of the colonies might be relied upon, but that they were unable to send delegates to the proposed congress because of the influence of Governor Wright. From this time forward the people became excited, which was more apparent as the time drew near for the act to go into force. An occasion for the manifestation of this spirit came on the 26th of October, 1765, which was the anniversary of the accession of his Majesty King George III to the throne of England. In honor thereof the Governor ordered a general muster in Savannah. This caused the assembling of a large number of people, who paraded effigies of obnoxious personages through the streets and then burned them.

The act was to take effect on the first of November, 1765, but the stamps did not arrive until the fifth of December, when they were transferred to Fort Halifax, for fear the "Liberty Boys" would destroy them, as they were pledged to do, and also to force the Agent to resign. The "Liberty Boys," two hundred strong, assembled around Fort Halifax on the second of January, 1766, and threatened to break open the fort and destroy the papers. This demonstration alarmed the Governor, but he determined to save the papers, and mustering the two companies of royal rangers marched to the fort, took out the stamps, and carried them in a cart to the guard-house. The people looked sullenly on but made no attempt to take the papers. The Governor was so alarmed for his personal safety that he kept a guard of forty men around his house and for four nights did not undress.* The day after the removal of the stamps Mr. Agnus, the stamp distributor, arrived off Tybee, of which, by preconcerted signals, the Governor was notified, and, fearing that the citizens would injure Agnus, had him secretly brought up to his garrisoned mansion, where a fortnight's residence convinced Agnus that his person was not safe, and caused him to leave town. Toward the close of January about six hundred armed men, a large number of whom were from Savannah, assembled near the town and sent word to the Governor that if the obnoxious papers were not removed they would come into town and destroy them, if they had to storm his house and the fort to accomplish their purpose. The Governor had the papers removed to Fort George, on Cockspur island. The next day two or three hundred men assembled on the commons and demanded a redress of their grievances. Governor Wright ordered out his marines and rangers, and for a time a conflict was imminent, but the people dispersed after burning an effigy of the Governor.

At the time of these troubles Savannah consisted of four hundred dwelling-houses, a church, an independent meeting-house, a council house, a court-house, and a filature. There were twelve streets besides the Bay, six squares, and two suburbs: Yamacraw on the west and the Trustees' garden on the east. The limits of the town on the east was what is now Lincoln street, on the west what is now Jefferson street, and on the south what is now South Broad street. When the stamps arrived there were between sixty and seventy sail in port waiting to be cleared, and the people consented that stamps might be used for this but no other purpose. This

* The Governor's house was situated on St. James square, fronting east on the lot where now stands the "Telfair honse," between State and President streets.

was done and the port opened, yet all judicial business was suspended and the courts closed.

This act gave great offence to the other colonies, and especially to South Carolina, the people of which colony resolved that no "provisions should be shipped to that infamous colony; that whosoever should traffic with them should be put to death; that every vessel trading there should be burnt;" and as a proof that these were not idle threats, two vessels on their way to Savannah, a short time after these threats were made, were seized before clearing Charleston bar and, with their cargoes, destroyed.

The repeal of the Stamp act, on the 22d of February, 1766, the announcement of which was received in Savannah on the sixth of July following, restored order and the people resumed their usual avocations and pursuits, which had been interrupted by the recent troubles.

The acts of the British Parliament in regard to duties upon imported goods, which were found "grievous to be borne," was the topic of the day in Savannah as well as everywhere else in the colonies of North America, and on the 16th of September, 1769, the merchants of Savannah met at the house of Alexander Creighton and resolved that

> Any person or persons whatsoever importing any of the articles subject to such duties, after having it in their power to prevent it, ought not only to be treated with contempt, but deemed as an enemy to their country—it being a circumstance that needs be only mentioned to any person inspired with the least sense of liberty that it may be detested and abhorred.

Governor Wright strenuously opposed every measure of the people that was in opposition to those of the British government, yet every one felt that he had faithfully discharged his duty to his king, and in such manner as to inspire respect and esteem from those who differed in sentiment; and upon his departure for England, on the tenth of July, 1771, just after dissolving the Assembly, the council, the bench, the merchants, and public officers presented him with addresses expressive of their respect and esteem. After his departure the gubernatorial mantle fell upon the shoulders of Mr. James Habersham, there to remain until the Governor's return, which occurred about the middle of February, 1773. During his absence the duties of the office were faithfully discharged by Mr. Habersham.

Governor Wright, on his arrival, found that the spirit of rebellion had increased; that the colony, and especially the people of Savannah, were in common with the rest of the colonists indignant at the closing of the port of Boston and divesting it of all commercial privileges. On the twentieth of July, 1774, those true and tried patriots, Noble Wimberly Jones, Archibald Bullock, John Houston, and George Walton, published a call in the Georgia Gazette for all persons within the limits of the province to attend at Tondee's tavern* on the 27th instant, to take under consideration the acts of the British Parliament, "which are particularly calculated to deprive the American subjects of their constitutional rights and liberties as parts of the British empire." A large number of persons assembled in pursuance of the call, but all of the parishes not being represented it was resolved to meet on the tenth of August, which was done, despite the proclamation of Governor Wright that the people should not assemble, and if they did it would be "at their peril." The meeting adopted resolutions protesting against the oppressive acts of Parliament and agreeing to concur with the sister colonies in every constitutional measure to obtain redress of American grievances. The citizens of Savannah who were most zealous in these acts of patriotism were: John Glenn, John Smith, Joseph Clay, John Houston, N. W. Jones, Lyman Hall, William Young, E. Telfair, Samuel Farley, George Walton, Joseph Habersham, Jonathan Bryan, Jonathan Cochrane, George W. McIntosh, — Sutton, William Gibbons, Benjamin Andrew, John Winn, John Stirk, A. Powell, James Beaven, D. Zubly, H. L. Bourquine, Elisha Butler, William Baker, Parmenus Way, John Baker, John Mann, John Bennefield, John Stacy, and John Morell.

A provincial congress, upon invitation of a committee of citizens of Christ Church parish, assembled in Savannah on the eighteenth of January, 1775, and elected John Glenn chairman. The congress was in session six days, and elected Noble Wimberly Jones, Archibald Bulloch, and John Houston delegates to represent Georgia in the Continental Congress, which assembled in Philadelphia on the 10th of May following. The delegates did not attend, but sent a letter, written on the 8th of April, 1775, stating that they could not call the proceedings of the congress which elected them the voice of the province, as but five out of twelve parishes were represented; that they found the inhabitants of

---

* Tondee's tavern was situated on the northwest corner of Broughton and Whitaker streets.

Savannah not likely soon to give matters a favorable turn; that the importers were mostly against any interruption, and the consumers here and elsewhere very much divided; that there were some of the latter virtually for the measures of resistance; others strenuously against them, but more who called themselves neutrals than either; they (the delegates) therefore did not attend, because the inhabitants of the province for which they would have appeared had refused to make any sacrifice to the public cause, and in whose behalf they did not think they could pledge themselves for the execution of any one measure whatsover.

Thus undecided and almost in a state of apathy did the major portion of the inhabitants of Savannah stand, while the people of the towns in other colonies were in a state of almost frantic excitement. But this indecision and apathy was of short duration. The tidings of the affray between the colonists and the British troops at Lexington, Massachusetts, reached Savannah on the night of the 10th of May, 1775, and caused great excitement among all classes, and all ideas of submission to British rule vanished. The following night Noble Wimberly Jones, Edward Telfair, Joseph Habersham, John Milledge, William Gibbons, and Joseph Clay seized the king's magazine, located where the gas-house now stands, and took therefrom five hundred pounds of powder and stored it in their cellars and garrets. The next day the Governor missed the powder, and by advice of the Council £150 reward was offered to any one who would give information which would lead to the arrest of those engaged in the seizure. Though all engaged were well known, no one gave the desired information. A large quantity of this powder was sent North, and it is asserted was used by the militia in the defence of Bunker Hill.

On Monday, the 5th day of June, the birthday of his Majesty King George III, the citizens, amid great rejoicing, raised a liberty pole (the first one raised in Georgia) in front of Tondee's public house. A Union flag was hoisted upon the pole and two pieces of artillery placed at the foot. A dinner was given immediately after the pole-raising, at which the first toast was "The King," and the second "American Liberty."

A meeting of the citizens was held at the residence of Mrs. Cuyler* on the 13th of June, at which were present John Mullryne,

* Located at the southeast corner of Bull and Broughton streets.

Joseph Clay, James Mossman, Rev. J. J. Zubly, John Simpson, Noble Wimberly Jones, John Jamieson, William Moss, John Glenn, Josiah Tatnall, John Graham, Lewis Johnston, William Young, Richard Wylly, Andrew McLean, Basil Cowper, Phillip Moore, George Houston, Joseph Butler, James Read, Thomas Reid, William Panton, James E. Powell, William Struthers, Alexander McGowan, John C. Lucena, Thomas Sherman, J. N. Faning, Levi S. Sheftall, Charles Hamilton, George Spencer, William Brown, jr., Francis Courvoizie, and James Anderson. John Mullryne was chosen president, and a number of resolutions adopted expressive of their feelings in regard to the existing troubles, among which were:

That we will use our utmost endeavors to preserve the peace and good order of this province; that no person behaving himself peaceably and inoffensively shall be molested in his personal property, or even in his private sentiments while he expresses them with decency and without any illiberal reflections upon others; that the interest of this province is inseperable from the mother country and the sister colonies, and that to separate ourselves from the latter would be only throwing difficulties in the way of its own relief and that of the other colonies, and justly increasing the resentment of all those to whose distress our disunion might be an addition; that this province ought, and it is hoped will, forthwith join the other provinces in every just and legal measure to secure and restore the liberties of all America; that these proceedings be laid before the Provincial Congress to meet on the 4th of July.

CHAPTER IV.

Organization of a Council of Safety — Meeting of the Provincial Congress — Capture of a British Vessel Loaded with Powder — Organization of a Batallion of Troops — Arrival of Two British Men-of-War off Tybee — Gallant Capture of Governor Wright by Major Joseph Habersham — Escape of the Governor — He Advises the People to Furnish Food to his Majesty's Ships — Attempt of the British to Capture Rice Ships in front of the Town — The People Resolve to Burn the Houses and Ships before they shall fall into the hands of the enemy — Repulse of the British — Reception of the Declaration of Independence and Burial of the Political Existence of George III—Adoption of the State Constitution—South Carolina Covets Savannah — Capture of the Town by the British.

On the 22d of June a Council of Safety, consisting of William Ewen, President; Seth John Cuthbert, Secretary; Joseph Habersham, Edward Telfair, William LeConte, Basil Cowper, Joseph Clay, George Walton, John Glenn, Samuel Elbert, William Young, Elisha Butler, George Houston, John Smith, Francis H. Harris, and John Morel, was appointed.

The Provincial Congress met in Tondee's Long Room on the 4th of July, of which Archicald Bulloch was elected President and George Walton Secretary. Archicald Bulloch, Noble Wimberly Jones, Joseph Habersham, Jonathan Bryan, Ambrose Wright, William Young, John Glenn, Samuel Elbert, John Houston, Joseph Reynolds, John Smith, Oliver Bowen, John McClure, Edward Telfair, Thomas Lee, George Houston, William Ewen, John Martin, Rev. Dr. J. J. Zubly, William Bryan, Phillip Box, Philip Allman, William O'Bryan, Joseph Clay, and John Cuthbert were the members from the town and district of Savannah. After organizing, Congress adjourned to the meeting-house of Rev. Dr. Zubly, where he preached a sermon upon the "alarming state of American affairs," based on the words of St. James, ii, 12: "So speak ye, and so do as they that shall be judged by the law of liberty." The Dr. received the thanks of Congress for "the excellent sermon he preached before them." *

* Dr. Zubly first espoused the cause of liberty, and being very popular, influenced a very large number to support it. When matters became serious and war seemed inevitable, he changed his sentiments, and while in Philadel-

Congress being informed that forty armed men in barges, under command of Captains John Barnwell and Joyner, had been sent to the mouth of the Savannah river, by South Carolina, to capture a British ship which was on its way to Savannah, laden with powder for the use of the Royalists, offered them every assistance. A schooner was armed and placed under command of Captains Bowen and Joseph Habersham for the purpose of capturing a British armed schooner then in the river near town. On the approach of the Georgia schooner the British schooner put to sea and escaped. The Georgia schooner then laid off Tybee, near which were the two South Carolina barges. On the 10th of July the ship with the powder, commanded by Captain Maitland, was descried in the offing, sailing boldly in. Before getting in range of the Georgia schooner Maitland's suspicions were aroused, and he tacked and put out to sea. He was pursued by the schooner, and with the assistance of the South Carolinians his vessel was captured. On board were sixteen thousand pounds of powder, nine thousand pounds of which fell to Georgia. This schooner was the first commissioned American vessel, and made the first capture of the war.

The battalion of troops for the protection of Georgia was organized in Savannah on the 7th of January, 1776 by the appointment of Lachlan McIntosh Colonel, Samuel Elbert Lieutenant-Colonel, and Joseph Habersham Major. These appointments were made by the Council of Safety, which met every Monday at Tondee's Long Room, at 10 A. M., and at such other times as occasion required.

On the 12th of January two men-of-war and a transport laden with troops, under command of Majors Maitland and Grant, arrived

---

phia attending the Continental Congress as a representative of Georgia, commenced a treasonable correspondence with Governor Wright, posting him in regard to the movements of the Liberty party. This correspondence being discovered, he returned to Savannah and openly took sides against the Liberty party. His conduct was so obnoxious to the people that he was banished from the town in 1777, and half of his estate taken from him. After the capture of the town by the British he returned to his ministerial charge and remained during the siege. He died on the 23d of July, 1781, at the age of fifty-six, broken in heart and broken in fortune, yet nobly struggling against misfortune, aiming to be faithful in the discharge of his ministerial duties and earnestly laboring to enter into that rest which remains for the people of God. Savannah still bears the record of this learned man in the names of two of its streets, "Joachim" and "Zubly;" and one of the hamlets was named St. Gall, in honor of his birth-place in Switzerland.—*Condensed from the account in the History of Georgia, by Right Reverend William Bacon Stevens.*

off Tybee. A meeting of the Council of Safety was called on the 18th, when it was resolved "that the persons of his Excellency Sir James Wright, Bart., and of John Mullryne, Josiah Tatnall, and Anthony Stokes, Esqs., be forthwith arrested and secured, and that all non-associates be forthwith disarmed, except those who will give their parole, assuring that they will not aid, assist, or comfort any of the persons on board his Majesty's ships-of-war, or take up arms against America in the present unhappy state of affairs." Major Joseph Habersham, who was then only twenty-four years of age, volunteered to secure the Governor. That evening while the Governor was in consultation with the Council at his house, Habersham proceeded thither alone, passed the sentinels at the door, entered the hall in which the Council was assembled, walked boldly up to the head of the table, and laying his hand upon the Governor's shoulder said: "Sir James, you are my prisoner." This bold act astonished the members of the Council, who, supposing from Habersham's firm manner he had a large force near by, fled precipitately through the doors and windows. The Governor gave his solemn parole that he would not go out of town or hold any communication with the British at Tybee, and was allowed to remain in his house under guard. Here he remained until the 11th of February, when, becoming weary of the confinement, the insults to which he was subjected by thoughtless persons, and also fearing that he would be killed by some of the many musket-balls fired into the house by the guards for amusement, he eluded the sentinels and ran to Bonaventure, escaping from thence in a small boat, furnished by John Mullryne, to the British ship Scarborough, on board of which he was received at three o'clock on the morning of the 12th. The following day the Governor wrote a letter to the members of his Council, all of whom had given the required parole, desiring it to be laid before the Provincial Congress. In this letter he, among other things, stated:

> Such is my regard for the people of Georgia that I can not avoid exhorting them to save themselves and their posterity from the total ruin and destruction which, although they may not, I most clearly see at the threshold of their doors, and I can not leave them without again warning them in the most earnest and friendly manner to desist from their present plans and resolutions. * * * * I have the great satisfaction to be able to affirm, from the best authority, that the forces now here will not commit any hostilities against this Province, although fully sufficient to reduce and overcome every opposition that could be attempted to be made; and that nothing is meant or wanted but a friendly intercourse and a supply of provisions. This his Majesty's

officers have an undoubted right to effect and what they insist upon, and this I not only solemnly require, in his Majesty's name, but also as (probably) the best friend the people of Georgia have, advise them, without the least hesitation, to comply with; or it may not be in my power to insure them the continuance of the peace and quietude they now have, if it may be called so.

The request for provisions was promptly refused, and Captain Barclay, commanding the British vessels, being very much in need, determined to capture the eleven rice ships which lay under the bluff awaiting an opportunity to run out to sea. Acccordingly, on the last day of February, 1776, the Scarborough, Hinchinbrooke, and St. John, with two transports laden with troops, sailed up to Five-fathom Hole, opposite the point on which Fort Jackson now stands.

Anticipating a speedy attack, the Council of Safety met on the 2d of March and appointed Messrs. Joseph Clay, Joseph Reynolds, John McClure, Joseph Dunlap, and John Glenn a committee "to value and appraise the houses in town and hamlets thereunto belonging, together with the shipping in the port, the property of or appertaining to the friends of America who have associated and appeared, or who shall appear in the present alarm to defend the same; and also the houses of the widows and orphans, and none others." It was also resolved to defend the town "so long as it was tenable, and that rather than it should be held by the enemy it and the shipping in the port should be burned." The houses of those inimical to the American cause were not valued. When the resolutions were promulgated, they met the hearty approval of all classes excepting a small number who were friendly to the Royal cause.

After dark on the 2d two of the enemy's vessels sailed up Back river. The Scarborough anchored opposite the town and the Hinchinbrooke attempted to sail around Hutchinson's island with a view of coming down the Savannah river to the rice vessels. In this effort she ran aground on the west side of the island, and was unable to get off. The eleven rice vessels were laying under the bluff, but that evening, for some reason which was never fully ascertained but it was supposed that the captains had been bought with British gold, moved over near to the Hutchinson island shore opposite Yamacraw. Every preparation for resisting the enemy was made by Colonel Lachlan McIntosh, acting under orders of the Council of Safety. Suspecting the captains, and fearing that they might be induced to run their vessels out to sea, he ordered Captain

Rice to go aboard of the vessels early the next morning and order the rudders and rigging to be sent on shore. The fort on the lower end of the bluff was strengthened and reinforced, and was deemed sufficiently powerful to repulse any attempt of the enemy to advance up the river. Major Habersham was ordered to take two companies of riflemen and proceed up the river opposite to the Hinchinbrooke and be ready to fire upon her at early dawn.

During the night about three hundred British soldiers landed on Hutchinson's island from the vessels in Back river and marched across and took possession of the rice vessels. This was done so quietly that the Americans knew nothing of it. Early on the 3d Captain Rice went over in a small boat to deliver the order given him and was taken prisoner. Two sailors were allowed by Majors Maitland and Grant, commanding the troops aboard of the rice vessels, to come over to town to get some clothing which they said had been left, they agreeing to go and return without communicating any information regarding the operations on the island side of the river. They were not true to their promise. They not only did not return, but told the Americans that the British had possession of the vessels and had captured Captain Rice. This was astounding news to the Americans and created intense excitement. All of the males were immediately mustered under arms, and three hundred men under Colonel McIntosh proceeded to Yamacraw and threw up a breastwork and placed three four-pounders in position.* Before this the riflemen under Habersham opened fire upon the Hinchinbrooke, which had floated off and was making another attempt to sail down. The tide was low and she made slow progress; besides this, the fire from the riflemen so galled the crew that they were driven below and did not attempt to manage the vessel. She was armed with twenty-eight guns; and at intervals the crew manned them and endeavored, by a free use of grape, to drive off their assailants, but of no avail. The riflemen protected themselves and fired with such accuracy as to kill and wound a number of the crew, and finally caused them to desist from their object. The lack of boats, only, prevented the riflemen from boarding and capturing her. Only one rifleman was injured by her fire, a small shot having struck him in the thigh.

Meanwhile the people and soldiers in town became clamorous

* Tradition asserts that "Battle Row," located on the bluff at the corner of West Broad street, is on the site of this breastwork.

for the rescue of Rice. Lieutenant Daniel Roberts, of the St. Johns Rangers, and Mr. Raymond Demere (afterward promoted to the rank of Major), of St. Andrew's parish, requested and were granted permission to go over and demand the surrender of the captain. They left their weapons and were rowed over by a negro. They landed on one of the vessels, aboard of which were Majors Grant and Maitland and Captain Barclay. They stated the object of their mission. The British officers, without making any reply, placed them under arrest. The Americans awaited nearly an hour for the return of their deputies and then called through trumpets to the British to know why they were detained. The British returned insulting replies; whereupon two cannon-shots were fired at them. This had the effect of making them send a letter over, signed by Roberts and Demere, stating that the enemy "would treat with any two people the Americans confided in." Without waiting for the action of the authorities, Captain Screven, of the St. Johns Rangers, and Captain Baker, of the St. Johns Riflemen, with about a dozen riflemen, rowed over to the Captain Inglis and peremptorily demanded the surrender of Rice, Roberts, and Demere. The officer commanding the vessel made an insulting reply, and received a rifle-shot from Captain Baker. The enemy immediately opened upon the boat with cannon and musketry. The riflemen also fired, at the same time hauling off. Their friends on the bluff, observing this attack upon a few men and also the perilous position they were in, opened on the vessels. A general engagement ensued, lasting four hours, during which no one was hurt on the American side, excepting a rifleman in the boat, who was wounded in the shoulder by the first fire from the vessel. At four o'clock the Council of Safety met and resolved to have the vessels across the river burned. Captain Bowen was ordered by Colonel McIntosh to attend to this duty. He, assisted by Lieutenants James Jackson and John Morel, took the Inverness, which lay on this side of the river laden with rice and deer skins, and set fire to her. She drifted across to the rice vessels and communicated the fire to some of them. The enemy, however, did not wait for her approach, but left the vessels and ran into the marsh in laughable confusion. The Americans fired upon them and killed and wounded a great number. The crews of two of the vessels remained on board and managed to escape the fire-vessel and sailed up the river under protection of the men-of-war. Six were destroyed by the fire and three saved from the flames and brought over to the town side. The British sailed down to Tybee the next day, carrying with them Rice, Roberts, and Demere. In order to recover them, the Council of Safety seized all members of the Royal Council then in Savannah and offered them in exchange. The offer was accepted, and on the 27th of March the prisoners were restored to their friends.

On the 8th of August the Declaration of Independence was received in Savannah, and was promulgated on the 11th by Archibald Bulloch, President of the Executive Committee of Georgia, in front of the Assembly Rooms, at the Liberty Pole, and at the battery. The troops were paraded and a salute of thirteen guns was fired after each reading. Late in the day a dinner was partaken of by the soldiers and citizens, after which a funeral procession was formed—the soldiers with arms reversed and muffled drums—and marched to the front of the court-house, where the political existence of George III was interred, the following funeral discourse being delivered:

> Forasmuch as George III, of Great Britain, hath most flagrantly violated his coronation oath, and trampled upon the constitution of our country and the sacred rights of mankind, we therefore commit his political existence to the ground—corruption to corruption—tyranny to the grave—and oppression to eternal infamy, in the sure and certain hope that he will never obtain a resurrection to rule again over these United States of America. But, my friends and fellow-citizens, let us not be sorry, as men without hope, for TYRANTS that thus depart—rather let us remember America is free and independent; that she is, and will be, with the blessing of the Almighty, GREAT among the nations of the earth. Let this encourage us in well-doing, to fight for our rights and privileges, for our wives and children, for all that is near and dear unto us. May God give us his blessing and all the people say AMEN.

A few days after the celebration a convention met in Savannah to form a State constitution, which was done. It was adopted on the 5th of February, 1777.

In January of 1777 William H. Drayton, who had been sent by the Assembly of South Carolina to treat with the Georgia Congress of an union between Georgia and South Carolina, which the Assembly of the latter province had resolved "would tend effectually to promote their strength, wealth, and dignity, and to secure their liberty, independence, and safety," arrived in Savannah, "and found," as he afterward wrote, "every gentleman in public office was strongly against an union," but a number of "gentlemen of fortune, not in office or convention, who heartily approved the measure." The advantages which would accrue to Savannah were nearly altogether spoken of by the Commissioner before the Convention, and led many to believe that the annexation of Savannah with South Carolina was more desired than the rest of the province. The Commissioner thus spoke:

The town of Savannah in particular, and the adjacent lands, would be of much more importance and value, because Savannah river would be immediately cleared, a measure that would encourage and occasion an immense increase of agriculture upon all land within reach of its navigation, and hence an amazing increase of produce and river navigation, all of which would centre in Savannah. Thus, in a state of separation from South Carolina, Savannah could reasonably expect, and that but by slow degrees, and at a distant day, only the one half of the produce of a well-improved cultivation of the lands on the Savannah river, but by an union she would, in a very short time, receive the whole of that improved cultivation and trade, and her own commerce would be increased almost beyond imagination, although she would lose the seat of government. Finally, I may add, that in a state of separation, in all probability, Savannah will be ruined, because it will be our interest to preserve our trade to our own people. A town will rise on the Carolina side of the Savannah river, which will be sure to preserve our half of the trade of that river, and by being wisely supported it may draw to it the other half also; and let it not be said, we can not find a situation for a town, because it ought to be remembered that history is full of instances of towns having been built and made to flourish in situations that had been deemed impracticable for such purposes. Rivers and lands make wealthy towns, for these are natural causes; the presence and expense of a few officers of Government are but drops of water in the ocean; these go but a little way toward filling a Government port with loaded ships. The principal materials for the building of such towns are policy and opulence; I thank God, Carolina is not known to be in want of either.

The proposed annexation was refused.* No town has risen to compete with Savannah, but the trade and commerce which was coveted has increased, the town has prospered, and now ranks the first city in beauty, and in point of wealth, refinement, and commerce among the first cities of the United States.

In the fall of 1778 Colonel McIntosh, who had been left in command of the town after the repulse of the British in March, 1776, notified General Robert Howe, commander of the American forces in this section, with headquarters at Charleston, that an advance of the enemy upon Savannah was anticipated, and that his small

* Notwithstanding the refusal, Drayton endeavored, by speeches and other methods, to influence the people in favor of the project. This he continued for some time, when Governor Treutlen offered a reward for his apprehension. Fearing an arrest he fled the State.

force, two hundred and fifty men, with one hundred for duty, was inadequate to defend the place. General Howe came over and took command. He had about five hundred regulars and three hundred and fifty militia. He learned that the enemy had planned for Colonel Prevost to advance from Florida and arrive near Savannah in time to co-operate with the fleet under Sir Hyde Parker and the troops under Lieutenant-Colonel Campbell, to be sent from New York. Prevost advanced as far as Sunbury. The Americans made a show of being in strong force and Prevost retreated. Howe then returned to Savannah and ordered all of the troops to assemble there. The town was in an almost defenseless condition, excepting from the water side. The fort on the eastern end of the bluff, where the gas-house now stands, had been considerably enlarged, more guns mounted, and made quite formidable. It was named Fort Wayne, in honor of General Anthony Wayne.

By the 27th of December the whole of the British fleet had anchored off Tybee. The vessels composing the armed squadron were the Phœnix, forty-four guns; the Rose and Fowey, twenty-four guns each; the Vigilant, twenty-eight guns; and the brig Keppel, the sloop Greenwich, and the galley Comet. The transports brought about thirty-five hundred men. Howe had about nine hundred men to oppose their force. The British were not at first aware of the weakness of the Americans, and were disposed to wait the arrival of Prevost's command before commencing the assault upon the town. To gain information Colonel Campbell sent a boat's crew ashore to capture some of the inhabitants. The crew landed on Wilmington island and took two men prisoners, who informed them of the exact condition of the Americans. Believing the information received to be correct, Campbell decided to attack without delay. On the 28th the squadron sailed up within two miles of town, opposite to Girardeau's plantation, and preparations were made to land early the next morning.

Howe was not correctly informed concerning the strength of the enemy, and believing he could cope with them, determined to defend the town. Observing this movement of the enemy, he rightly concluded that the troops would land below Brewton hill* and advance upon the town by the great road, now known as the Thunderbolt road, and Captain John C. Smith, with his com-

* This hill is about a mile and a half in a direct line below the city, on the plantation of T. F. Screven.

pany of South Carolinians, was sent to the hill to watch the enemy. The marsh on the east side of the city was then much wider and more difficult to cross than now. On the high ground west of the marsh General Howe placed his command so as to cover the great road, which crossed the marsh by a narrow causeway, and burned the bridge over the rivulet which ran through the centre of the marsh. To present still further obstructions, a deep ditch was dug three hundred yards west of the marsh and filled with water. The army was divided into two brigades; the first, commanded by Colonel Elbert, constituted the left, and the other, under Colonel Huger, the right wing.* Five pieces of cannon were posted in front of the causeway. To the right of the position of the Americans a small path led through the swamp to the high grounds on the opposite side. This path was pointed out to General Howe by Colonel Walton as a place which should be guarded, but the General, thinking differently, paid no attention to the suggestion. About what is now the corner of Liberty and Bull streets were the New barracks. The roads to White Bluff and the Ogeechee river united near the barracks, and Colonel Walton, with one hundred militia, was posted there.

About dawn of the 29th the British landed on Girardeau's place. From the point of landing to Brewton's hill was a narrow causeway six hundred yards in length. A body of Highlanders, under Captain Cameron, landed first and were thrown forward to secure the hill. Captain Smith ordered his men to reserve their fire until the enemy were close. The Highlanders marched in solid column half-way up the hill, when the Americans opened upon them, killing Captain Cameron and two privates, and wounding five others. The first and second battalions of DeLancy's corps of New York Volunteers and the first battalion of the 71st regiment of foot, all under Lieutenant-Colonel Maitland, had landed immediately after the Highlanders, and hearing the firing rushed forward to participate. The Highlanders, who had been thrown into confusion by the effective fire of the Americans, rallied and advanced with their reinforcement. Captain Smith, who had been instructed to retire if attacked by a large force, retreated

---

* The exact position of the American line on the southeast of the city is not known, but it is supposed to have been stretched across the road to Thunderbolt, a short distance west of what is now the site of the Atlantic and Gulf Railroad depot.

to the main body. The entire force of the enemy now landed and formed line-of-battle on top of the hill and there remained, while Colonel Campbell with a small party rode forward to reconnoitre. This done, the light infantry, under Sir James Baird, were thrown forward, supported by DeLancy's New York Volunteers. Following these came the first battalion of the 71st with two six-pounders, and Wellworth's battalion of Hessians, with two three-pounders. By three o'clock the army arrived within eight hundred yards of the Americans and halted. The advantageous position selected by General Howe was duly noted and appreciated by Colonel Campbell, and he determined that no benefits should be derived from it, and therefore aimed to turn Howe's right flank or get into his rear. In his reconnoisances he ran across an old negro named Quanimo Dolly, generally called Quash, who informed him of the private path through the swamp, by which the rear of the American line could be gained. Overjoyed at this discovery, Campbell returned to his command and ordered Sir James Baird, with the light infantry and the New York Volunteers, to follow the negro through the swamp and attack the first body of troops found. To deceive the Americans, Colonel Campbell manœuvred his troops in front as if about to attack. This caused the Americans to play upon them with their artillery. The British did not return the fire, but still manœuvred, waiting to hear from Baird. He followed the negro through the swamp, coming out at a point near where is now Waringsville, and struck the White Bluff road, down which he advanced, falling suddenly upon the small force of Walton's. This was swept away after a short but brave resistance, during which Walton was wounded, and the conqueror turned to the right to strike the rear of the American line. The firing notified Campbell that Baird had accomplished his purpose, and he immediately advanced his line at a rapid pace. The artillery, which had been concealed behind a hill, was pushed forward to the top and a rapid fire opened upon the Americans. Sir James Baird also charged from the rear. The Americans were between two fires, and opposed to them was a force much larger and better disciplined. Nothing but a retreat was now left to them. The order was given for Colonel Daniel Roberts, with the artillery, to secure the causeway on the Augusta road leading across Musgrove creek and swamp, on the west of the town. This he did, and the right flank retreated to it and crossed in safety. The left flank attempted to retreat by this route, but before their arrival the British drove Colonel Roberts across the causeway and took possession. Colonel Elbert's command, many of whom had been shot and bayonetted as they ran through town, finding this avenue of retreat denied them, rushed through the rice-fields near the river. The tide was up and Musgrove creek full of water. A large number threw away their arms and accoutrements and attempted to swim it. Most of them succeeded, but thirty of the number were drowned. The remainder of the command, two hundred in number, either could not swim or dared not attempt to cross and there stopped, to be captured a few moments after. These were marched back to town, disarmed, and robbed by the Highlanders. Sir James Baird coming up at the time with others of the Highlanders "mounted himself on a ladder and sounded his brass bugle-horn, which the Highlanders no sooner heard than they all got about him, when he addressed himself to them in Highland language, when they all dispersed and finished plundering such of the officers and men as had been fortunate enough to escape the first search." *

During the attack by the army the British fleet was made ready for action, and as soon as it was ascertained that the American line had given way Sir Hyde Parker sailed up the river and passed Fort Wayne, receiving a few shots therefrom, which killed and wounded five seamen. The galley Comet was sent further up the river and prevented any of the American vessels from escaping; thus securing to the squadron three ships, three brigs, and three smaller vessels, and one hundred and twenty-six prisoners. The army captured thirty-eight officers, four hundred and fifteen non-commissioned officers and privates, one stand of colors, forty-eight cannon, twenty-three mortars, six hundred and thirty-seven stand of arms, ninety barrels of powder, and other munitions of war; all done with the loss of only one commissioned officer and three men killed and one sergeant and fourteen men wounded. The Americans lost eighty-three men killed, thirty drowned, and a large number wounded.

The conduct of the British troops upon entering the town was of such a character as to strike terror to the hearts of all the inhabitants. Before the soldiers could be restrained lawless and brutal acts were committed; women were insulted, citizens who

---

* From the account of the capture of Mordecai Sheftall, Deputy Commissary-General of Issues to the Continental troops.

had not been engaged in the fight shot and bayonetted in the streets, and a number seized and carried aboard the ships, where they endured the most terrible sufferings from lack of food, pure air, and water. Among those thus imprisoned were the Honorable Jonathan Bryan, his son James, Reverend Moses Allen, Mordecai Sheftall, and his son Sheftall Sheftall, Edward Davis, Dr. George Wells, and David Moses Vallaton.

The remnant of Howe's army retreated up the river to Zubly's ferry and crossed into South Carolina. Campbell left Lieutenant-Colonel Innis in command of Savannah and marched to Augusta, shortly after which Brevet Brigadier-General Prevost arrived and relieved Colonel Innis. General Prevost established his head-quarters at the house situated on the north side of Broughton street next east of the Masonic hall.

CHAPTER V.

Treatment of the Inhabitants by the British — Plans of the Americans and French to Recapture the Town — Appearance of the French Troops under Count d'Estaing before the Town—Correspondence between Count d'Estaing and General Prevost regarding the Surrender of the Town—Arrival of the Americans — The British Reinforced — Commencement of Hostilities — Bombardment of the Town by the Allies — Women and Children Killed — Houses Demolished — Progress of the Siege — Unparalleled Act of Heroism — Women and Children not allowed to leave town during the Siege — Assault upon Spring Hill Redoubt by the Besiegers — They are Repulsed with heavy loss—Count Pulaski and Count d'Estaing wounded—Sergeant Jasper mortally wounded while bearing off the Colors of his Regiment — Abandonment of the Siege — Death and Burial of Count Pulaski.

The British rule was most stringent and exacting, subjecting the inhabitants to every manner of annoyance. A reward of two guineas was offered for every citizen that adhered to the American cause and ten guineas for every committeeman or assemblyman that should be delivered up to the king's officers. All articles of merchandise, country produce, and market vegetables had to be sold at fixed prices, and only by those who had taken the oath of allegiance; if these rules were violated the articles were confiscated, and if the trader sold to any other than loyal persons he was fined two hundred pounds. Those who remained true to the cause of liberty were, consequently, dependent upon the charity of those who had taken the oath. Their sufferings were almost beyond endurance, but had to be borne uncomplainingly, for the least murmur of complaint was reported to headquarters by spies, and the complainant arrested, subjected to insult, and in most instances deprived of his property by confiscation.* These persecutions were borne without a hope of relief until the fall of 1779, when the people were overjoyed by the appearance of a French fleet and army and the American army near the town, which they thought would recapture the town and relieve them from the oppressors.

* A number of ladies who openly avowed their sentiments were confined to their houses under guard, and Mrs. Judy Minis and her mother were ordered to leave town.

General Howe, shortly after his defeat here, was relieved by General Benjamin Lincoln. Early in 1778 a treaty was effected between France and the United States, and common cause was made against the British. The French government sent a large fleet and a small army over, under Count d'Estaing, to co-operate with the Americans. A plan for the capture of the British army in Philadelphia by the combined armies failed, owing to a storm which prevented the fleet from arriving in time. Count d'Estaing then sailed to the West Indies and captured two towns, Grenada and St. Vincent. While there General Lincoln, through the French Consul, solicited his co-operation in a proposed attempt to recapture Savannah. Count d'Estaing agreed to the plan, and it was arranged for the combined forces to appear in front of the town on the 17th of September, 1779.

On the 3d of September Count d'Estaing's fleet arrived off Tybee, the fleet consisting of twenty line-of-battle and two fifty-gun ships, eleven frigates, and five small armed vessels, with five thousand soldiers. The arrival was utterly unexpected by the British, and a portion of their fleet, under Sir James Wallace (son-in-law of Governor Wright), was captured. Colonel Joseph Habersham, who had been instructed by General Lincoln to meet Count d'Estaing at Tybee and make arrangements for the disembarkation of the French, effected an interview on the 11th, when it was decided to land the following night. Accordingly, shortly after dark the troops were placed in small vessels and conveyed to Beaulieu (the old seat of President William Stephens), about twelve miles from Savannah, and by the 15th all of the troops were landed at this place and intrenching tools sent ashore at Thunderbolt. General Lachlan McIntosh and Count Casimir Pulaski marched from Augusta and swept the enemy's advanced guards out of the way, capturing and killing some and driving the others into town. General McIntosh then fell back about three miles from town and Count Pulaski marched to Beaulieu, effecting a junction with Count d'Estaing on the 15th. The following day the line of march was taken up for Savannah, in front of which they arrived at noon.

Meanwhile the British had not been idle. The arrival of the French fleet was communicated to General Prevost on the 4th of September. Anticipating that an attack upon the town was shortly intended, he ordered Lieutenant-Colonel Cruger, at Sunbury, and Lieutenant-Colonel Maitland, at Beaufort, to report with their commands. Some old redoubts thrown up as a protection against the indians, but which were considered so worthless and disadvantageously placed that the Americans fought outside of them when attacked by the British in 1778, had been repaired by the British and twenty-three guns placed in position previous to the arrival of the French fleet. A force of twelve hundred men, three hundred of whom were negroes, were set to work under the direction of Major Moncrief, constructing new works, mounting guns, and making other preparations to resist the apprehended attack. By the sixteenth, a chain of redoubts thirteen in number, mounting seventy-six guns and mortars, a number of which had been taken from the vessels, were thrown up. These redoubts extended from the river at a point a little east of what is now East Broad street to the New barracks,* thence diverged to what is now South Broad street, thence to where the Central Railroad depot and workshops now stand. This point was then known as Spring Hill, and was the best fortified position on the lines, and commanded the road to Ebenezer and Augusta. The Musgrove creek and swamp on the west side of the city were almost impassable, and therefore only two small redoubts were thrown up on that side of the town. As a precautionary measure, the Germain was anchored off the mouth of the creek to rake the rice-fields along that stream. Prevost, fearing that the French frigates would sail close up to town and fire into the rear of his lines, sunk six vessels, the Fowey, Savannah, and four transports, across the channel below the town. Several small vessels were sunk above the town and a boom laid across the river to prevent fire-rafts from floating down the river among the shipping. On the 10th Colonel Cruger arrived, and with his forces aided in constructing the defences. In addition to the regular soldiers, Prevost had all of the sailors of the armed and merchant vessels posted at the guns; the three hundred negroes were also armed. All of these preparations were completed when d'Estaing arrived; yet Prevost was not satisfied that he could make a successful resistance without Maitland's troops, eight hundred in number, who were hourly expected, and desired to gain time.

We left d'Estaing a short distance from town on the 16th. His troops had hardly halted before he sent a pompous demand for the immediate surrender of the town, as follows:

* Near what is now the corner of Liberty and Bull streets.

Count d'Estaing summons his Excellency General Prevost to surrender to the arms of the King of France. He apprises him that he will be personally responsible for all the events and misfortunes that may arise from a defence, which by the superiority of the force that attacks him, both by sea and land, is rendered manifestly vain and of no effect.

He gives notice to him also, that any resolution he may venture to come to, either before the attack, in the course of it, or at the moment of the assault, of setting fire to the shipping, or small craft belonging to the army, or to the merchants in the river of Savannah, as well as to all the magazines in the town, will be imputable to him only.

The situation of Hospital hill in the Grenadas, the strength of the three intrenchments and stone redoubts which defended it, and the comparative disposition of the troops before the town of Savannah, with a single detachment which carried the Grenadas by assault, should be a lesson to futurity. Humanity obliges the Count d'Estaing to recall this event to his memory; having so done, he has nothing to reproach himself with.

Lord Macartney had the good fortune to escape from the first transport of troops who entered a town sword in hand, but notwithstanding the most valuable effects were deposited in a place supposed by all the officers and engineers to be impregnable, Count d'Estaing could not have the happiness of preventing their being pillaged. ESTAING.

Camp before Savannah, the 16th of September, 1779.

To this pompous demand General Prevost sent the following reply:

CAMP NEAR SAVANNAH, September 16, 1779.

SIR: I am just now honored with your Excellency's letter of this date, containing a summons for me to surrender this town to the arms of his Majesty the King of France; which I had just delayed to answer till I had shown it to the King's civil governor.

I hope your Excellency will have a better opinion of me, and of British troops, than to think either will surrender on general summons, without any specific terms.

If you, Sir, have any to propose, that may with honor be accepted of by me, you can mention them, both with regard to civil and military; and I will then give my answer. In the meantime I will promise, upon my honor, that nothing with my consent or knowledge shall be destroyed in either this town or river.

[Signed] A. PREVOST.

His Excellency Count d'Estaing, French forces, &c., &c.

To this Count d'Estaing replied:

CAMP BEFORE SAVANNAH, September 16th, 1779.

SIR: I have just received your Excellency's answer to the letter I had the honor of writing to you this morning. You are sensible that it is the part of the besieged to propose such terms as they may desire; and you can not doubt of the satisfaction I shall have in consenting to those which I can accept consistently with my duty.

5*

I am informed that you continue intrenching yourself. It is a matter of very little importance to me; however, for form's sake, I must desire that you will desist during our conferences.

The different columns which I had ordered to stop will continue their march, but without approaching your posts or reconnoitering your situation.

I have the honor to be, with respect, Sir, your Excellency's most humble and most obedient servant,

[Signed] ESTAING.

His Excellency General Prevost, Major-General in the service of his Britannic Majesty and Commander-in-Chief at Savannah, in Georgia.

P. S.—I apprise your Excellency that I have not been able to refuse the army of the United States uniting itself with that of the king.

The junction will probably be effected this day. If I have not an answer, therefore, immediately, you must confer in future with General Lincoln and me.

General Prevost replied:

CAMP NEAR SAVANNAH, September 16th, 1779.

SIR: I am honored with your Excellency's letter in reply to mine of this day.

The business we have in hand being of importance, there being various interests to discuss, a just time is absolutely necessary to deliberate. I am, therefore, to propose, that a suspension of hostilities shall take place for twenty-four hours from this date; and to request that your Excellency will order your columns to fall back to a greater distance and out of sight of our works, or I shall think myself under the necessity to direct their being fired upon. If they did not reconnoitre anything this afternoon they were sure within the distance.

[Signed] A. PREVOST.

His Excellency Count d'Estaing, &c., &c.

Count d'Estaing replied as follows, granting the request, yet intimating that he knew the cause of it:

CAMP BEFORE SAVANNAH, September 16th, 1779.

SIR: I consent to the truce you ask. It shall continue till the signal for retreat to-morrow night, the 17th, which will serve also to announce the recommencement of hostilities. It is unnecessary to observe to your Excellency that this suspension of arms is entirely in your favor, since I can not be certain that you will not make use of it to fortify yourself, at the same time that the propositions you shall make may be inadmissible.

I must observe to you, also, how important it is that you should be fully aware of your own situation as well as that of the troops under your command. Be assured that I am thoroughly acquainted with it. Your knowledge of military affairs will not suffer you to be ignorant that a due examination of that circumstance always precedes the march of the columns; and that this preliminary is not carried into execution by a mere show of troops.

I have ordered them to withdraw before night comes on, to prevent any cause of complaint on your part. I understand that my civility in this respect has been the occasion that the Chevalier de Chambis, a lieutenant in the navy, has been made a prisoner of war.

I propose sending out some small advanced posts to-morrow morning. They will place themselves in such a situation as to have in view the four entrances into the wood, in order to prevent a similar mistake in future. I do not know whether two columns, commanded by the Viscount de Noailles and the Count de Dillon, have shown too much ardor, or whether your cannoniers have not paid a proper respect to the truce subsisting between us; but this I know, that what has happened this night is a proof that matters will soon come to a decision between us one way or another.

I have the honor to be, with respect, &c.,

[Signed] ESTAING.

His Excellency General Prevost, Major-General in the service of his Britannic Majesty and Commander-in-Chief at Savannah, in Georgia.

The whole day was spent in the interchange of these notes, which resulted in Prevost's obtaining the time he so much desired. The following day General Lincoln arrived and held a council of war with d'Estaing, who informed him of what had transpired. General Lincoln was much displeased at the unseemly haste and lack of courtesy of d'Estaing, and so expressed himself.

During the interchange of notes between Prevost and d'Estaing Colonel Maitland was making all speed to join Prevost. His command, in small vessels, arrived in the river, during a dense fog, early on the 17th. The French squadron lay a little way up the river. An attempt to pass them would only have caused the destruction or capture of his command, and Maitland knew not what to do. Fortune and the ignorance of the commander of the French fleet favored him. A negro oystering near by was captured, and in response to interrogations concerning the channel informed Maitland that he knew of a way of reaching Savannah without passing in range of the guns of the fleet. The negro was pressed into service and piloted the vessels through Wall's cut* into the river above the hostile squadron. A few more moments and the troops were landed upon the bluff amid the cheers of the garrison, which now numbered twenty-eight hundred men. There were now one hundred and eighteen guns, including field pieces, in position, the redoubts were in order, the approaches to them protected by abattis, and a sufficient number of men to cope with the enemy. Prevost and his troops, before the arrival of Maitland, were

* In 1862 the Confederates failed to guard this cut. The Federal gun-boats passed through into the river and cut off communication between Fort Pulaski and the city.

depressed, believing the town would have to be surrendered; in fact, the incipient measures to that end had been taken. Now all were hopeful and the commander confident that he could make a successful resistance; and an hour after receiving the reinforcement addressed the following note to Count d'Estaing:

SAVANNAH, September 17, 1779,

SIR: In answer to the letter of your Excellency, which I had the honor to receive about twelve last night, I am to acquaint you that, having laid the whole correspondence before the King's civil governor and the military officers of rank assembled in council of war, the unanimous determination has been that, though we can not look upon our post as absolutely inexpugnable, yet that it may and ought to be defended; therefore, the evening-gun to be fired this evening at an hour before sundown shall be the signal for recommencing hostilities, agreeable to your Excellency's proposal.

I have the honor to be A. PREVOST.

The turn affairs had taken was entirely unanticipated, and the elation it occasioned among the British had a corresponding depressing influence among the allied forces. The opportunity for taking the town by assault, which could have been easily done on the 16th or early on the 17th, had passed. A siege was determined upon. As it was not anticipated that this would have to be done no preparations had been made for it; consequently, considerable delay ensued in procuring the requisite cannon, mortars, and ammunition from the French fleet.

A new work was begun by the British, on the night of the 21st, in front of the New barracks for six and nine-pounders. The walls of the barracks were also pulled down to within a few feet of the ground and the bricks thrown in front and on either side. These were covered with sand and dirt and a most formidable work made. This was done during the night. The besiegers, who had observed the building up to the night before and pointed it out as a good mark for their gunners, were much surprised the next morning not to see any trace of the building and to receive a severe fire of artillery from the spot where it stood only twelve hours before.

On the night of the 23d both the American and French armies broke ground together, about a mile from the enemy's works, the Americans on the left. On the night of the 24th a sap was pushed forward to within three hundred yards of the Spring Hill redoubt. At nine o'clock, A. M., on the 25th, Major Graham, of the 16th regiment, made a sortie for the purpose of reconnoitering the position of the allies. They dashed up to the sap and momentarily had possession of it. The French immediately dislodged the British and pursued them so ardently that they unexpectedly rushed under the guns of the British redoubts. The artillery was brought into play and the French fell back to the main line, with a loss of fifteen killed and thirty-five or forty wounded. The British lost seven killed and fifteen wounded.

The 25th and 26th were spent in harmless canonading and picket firing. At night on the 27th Major McArthur, of the 71st, sallied out to a small advanced work of the French, hoping to spike some cannon. He was discovered, and after firing a few rounds retreated unperceived. The French attempted to gain his left and the Americans his right flank. The advance of each party met, and each thinking the other the British, commenced a brisk fire. About fifty lives were lost before the mistake was discovered.

On the 28th the French frigate La Trinitie sailed up the Back river and anchored opposite the town. Two galleys at the same time moved up to the sunken vessels and fired upon the town, being joined by the frigate. The frigate was too far off, and her shots did no execution. The fire from the galleys injured several of the houses.

General Lachlan McIntosh on the 29th solicited and obtained permission from General Lincoln to send a flag-of-truce to General Prevost, requesting him to permit Mrs. McIntosh and children, and such other women and children as desired, to leave town during the siege. Major Jones bore the flag and found Mrs. McIntosh and children in a cellar, where they had been for six days. All of the cellars were crowded with the women and children. General Prevost, imagining that by retaining the women and children in town the besiegers would be restrained from throwing bombs and carcasses into it, refused to allow any one to leave.

During the night of the first of October, Colonel John White, with Captains George Melvin and A. G. Elholm and three soldiers, reconnoitred the position of Captain French, who, with five vessels, four of them fully armed, had attempted to sail up the Savannah river and reinforce Prevost, but the presence of the French fleet prevented and he sailed up the Ogeechee, intending to march his force of one hundred and thirty men over land. Arriving at a point about twenty miles from Savannah he ascertained that the Americans and French were between him and town. He concluded to await events and made a descent on shore, posting his men in an advantageous position, which was further protected by the vessels which were stationed so that they could aid in repelling an attack. Colonel White fully reconnoitred the position and formed the bold plan of capturing the men and vessels with his small force of five men. White gives an account of the affair in his "Historical Collections of Georgia," from which we extract it:

> The party then built a large number of watch-fires around the camp, placing them in such a position and at such intervals as to induce Captain French and his soldiers to believe that they were absolutely surrounded by a large force. The deception was kept up through the night by White and his companions, marching from fire to fire with the measured tread and the loud challenge of sentinels, now hailing from the east of the British camp, and then shifting rapidly their position and challenging from the extreme west. Nor was this the only stratagem; each mounted a horse and rode with haste in divers directions, imitating the manner of the staff, and giving orders with a loud voice. The delusion was complete. Captain French suffered himself to be completely trapped. White carried his daring plan forward by dashing boldly and alone to the camp of the British and demanding a conference with French. "I am commander, Sir," he said, "of the American soldiers in your vicinity. If you will surrender at once to my force, I will see to it that no injury is done to you or your command. If you decline to do this, I must candidly inform you that the feelings of my troops are highly incensed against you, and I can by no means be responsible for any consequences that may ensue." French thanked him for his humanity, and said, despondingly, that it was useless to contend with fate or with the large force that he saw was around him, and announced his willingness to surrender his vessels, his arms, his men, and himself to Colonel White. At this instant Captain Elholm came suddenly dashing up at full speed, and saluting White, inquired of him where he should place the artillery. "Keep them back, keep them back, Sir," answered White, "the British have surrendered. Move your men off, and send me three guides to conduct them to the American post at Sunbury." The three guides arrived. The five vessels were burned, and the British, urged by White to keep clear of his men, and to hasten their departure from the enraged and formidable Americans, pushed on with great celerity, whilst White retired with one or two of his associates, stating that he would go to his troops in the rear and restrain them. He now employed himself in collecting the neighborhood militia, with which he overtook his guides and conducted the prisoners in safety to the Sunbury post.

"The extraordinary address of White," says General Lee in his account of the affair, "was contrasted by the extraordinary folly of Captain French, and both were necessary to produce this wonderful issue. The affair approaches too near the marvelous to have been admitted into these memoirs, had it not been uniformly asserted as uniformly accredited and never contradicted."

The French frigate and galleys canonaded the left of the enemy's line on the third, which, says a British account, "had no other effect than to point out where to make traverses." At midnight of the same day the batteries of the allies opened fire on the town, continuing it until two o'clock, then ceasing, only to resume at daybreak, with thirty-seven guns and a number of mortars from the land side and sixteen guns from the frigate. The British batteries responded, and the canonading was kept up at intervals throughout the day, without much damage to the soldiers or works of either army, but missiles from the besiegers killed several women and children and three or four negroes. A young mother with an infant in her arms was lying on the bed in a house in the central part of the town, when a shell passed through, in its course killing both mother and child.

The fifth was passed in comparative quiet; but on the sixth the besiegers resumed the bombardment, which demolished several houses and burnt one. At eleven o'clock General Prevost sent the following request to Count d'Estaing:

CAMP SAVANNAH, October 6th, 1779.

SIR: I am persuaded that your Excellency will do me justice; and that in defending this place, and the army committed to my charge, I fulfil what is due to honor and duty to my prince. Sentiments of a different kind occasion the liberty of now addressing myself to your Excellency; they are those of humanity. The houses of Savannah are occupied solely by women and children. Several of them have applied to me, that I might request the favor you would allow them to embark on board a ship or ships, and go down the river under the protection of yours, until this business is decided. If this requisition you are so good as to grant, my wife and children, with a few servants, shall be the first to profit by this indulgence.

I have the honor to be, &c., &c. A. PREVOST.

As General Prevost had refused to grant a similar request made by the allies on the 29th, they refused to accede to this request, assigning their reasons therefor in the reply, which is as follows:

CAMP BEFORE SAVANNAH, October 6th, 1779.

SIR: We are persuaded that your Excellency knows all that your duty prescribes; perhaps your zeal has already interfered with your judgment. The Count d'Estaing, in his own name, notified to you that you would be personally and alone responsible for the consequences of your obstinacy. The time which you informed him, in the commencement of the siege, would be necessary for the arrangement of articles, including the different orders of men in your town, had no other object than that of receiving succor. Such conduct, Sir, is sufficient to forbid every intercourse between us which might occasion the least loss of time. Besides, in the present application, latent reasons may again exist. There are military ones, which in frequent instances have prevented the indulgence you request. It is with regret we yield to the austerity of our functions; and we deplore the fate of those persons who will be the victims of your conduct and the delusion which appears to prevail in your mind.

We are, with respect, &c., &c.,

[Signed] B LINCOLN.
ESTAING.

There was no cessation of hostilities during this correspondence; the bombardment was continued throughout the day, also on the seventh and eighth, neither besiegers nor besieged suffering materially from it. Early on the morning of the eighth, Captain l'Enfant with five men rushed up under a heavy fire to the abattis in front of the British works and attempted to burn it, but failed, owing to the greenness of the wood and the damp air. This was done to remove, if possible, these obstructions preparatory to an assault which had been determined upon. The Spring Hill redoubt was selected as the point to be attacked, and before dawn on the ninth as the time for the assault. On the 8th General Lincoln issued orders for the troops to be supplied with forty rounds of ammunition and to parade after midnight. Count d'Estaing was to lead the attack with the French, followed by Pulaski with his legion, which was ordered to penetrate the enemy's line between the Spring Hill redoubt and the next toward the river, then pass to the left into Yamacraw and secure all parties of the enemy in that quarter. The Americans under command of Colonel Laurens were to follow Pulaski. Count Dillon, with a small body of French, was to attack on the left of the Augusta road. Colonel Huger was to proceed around to the enemy's left with five hundred men and make an attack at four o'clock. This attack was only intended as a feint. Each soldier was forbidden to fire his weapon before the redoubt was carried; and to distinguish them from the enemy, each was ordered to wear a piece of white paper in his hat. It was also ordered that if the troops were repulsed after taking the Spring Hill redoubt they were to rally in rear of that redoubt; and if repulsed before taking it, to rally at the Jews' burying-ground.* The allies were confident of success and impatiently awaited the order for attack. During the night a sergeant-major of the Ameri-

---

* This burying-ground is still to be seen. It is in Robertsville, about six hundred yards in a southwesterly direction from the Central Railroad shops. Most of the walls are torn down. Another cemetery has been established about twenty paces distant, in which the Hebrews now inter their dead.

can grenadiers deserted to the enemy, carrying a copy of the order for the attack. General Prevost had expected an attack, but thought it would be made upon his left, which was more easily approached than any other portion of his line. Acting upon this information he reinforced the right of his line and assigned Colonel Graham to command there.

Unaware that their plan of attack was known to the enemy the allies moved forward to the assault, but owing to the darkness failed to reach the positions assigned them until daylight. The British were on the alert, and as soon as they were seen opened a heavy fire upon them. This was not anticipated, but, nothing daunted, the French pushed forward, followed by the Americans on the left. Both parties reached the redoubt and planted their flags upon it, but in a few moments were driven away, only to press forward again. The 2d South Carolina was foremost in the attack, and its standard was planted upon the work by Lieutenants Bush and Hume. They were almost instantly killed, and the colors fell with them into the ditch. Lieutenant Gray then seized them and once more they floated from the works, but he, too, was shot down. At his fall Sergeant Jasper rushed forward and bore them aloft, but human endurance could not withstand the terrific fire of the British and the Americans retreated, Sergeant Jasper carrying off the colors.* Count Dillon lost his way in Musgrove swamp, and early in the morning found himself exposed to the fire of the vessels off Musgrove creek and the redoubts in front. He endeavored to advance, but was speedily driven back. Count d'Estaing succeeded in effecting a lodgment on the left of the Spring Hill redoubt, but being wounded twice had to be carried off the field and his troops were thrown into disorder. Count Pulaski broke through the lines, as ordered, and was pushing forward, when he heard that d'Estaing was wounded and both the

---

* Sergeant Jasper greatly distinguished himself during the bombardment of Fort Moultrie by the British fleet some time previous. During the hottest part of the engagement the flag-staff was cut in two. Jasper caught the flag, seized a sponge-staff, and, tying the flag to it, jumped upon the ramparts and held it there until a new staff was procured. For this brave act he was offered a commission, but modestly refused to accept it, stating that he could neither read nor write, and therefore did not deem himself worthy; A short time after, his regiment (the 2d South Carolina) was presented with a stand of colors, beautifully embroidered, by Mrs. Elliott. Jasper received them, and swore to protect them with his life. Governor Rutledge at the same time presented him with a sword, and again offered him a commission, which he again refused.

Americans and French retreating. He left his command with Colonel Horry and galloped to the front of the retreating troops and bade them follow him. Animated by his brave example and cheering words, a large number turned and again advanced to the Spring Hill redoubt. A small cannon-shot struck Pulaski in the groin as he was entering the redoubt, and he fell from his horse. This discouraged the troops and they retreated, leaving Pulaski on the field. Hearing of this a large number of his legion advanced through the terrible fire and bore him to the rear. The British under Major Glasier followed the allies, but their retreat was so well covered by General Lincoln that the enemy took no prisoners and suffered considerably for their boldness. Colonel Huger made the feint on the left as ordered. The enemy were prepared, and received him with music and musket and cannon balls. He lost twenty-eight men and retreated.

The allies having lost a large number in killed and wounded were disspirited, and were glad to seek shelter behind their works, leaving the enemy complete masters of the situation. The conflict begun at daybreak and was over by nine o'clock, and at ten Prevost was requested to grant a truce to bury the dead and carry off the wounded, who were strewn in and on the works, in the ditch, and in front. Prevost granted a truce of four hours, stipulating that only those some distance from the works should be buried or cared for by their friends. Those of the dead near were buried by the British, and the wounded, one hundred and eighteen in number, sent over. The British lost over one hundred men during the siege, fifty-seven of whom were killed during the assault.* The combined army numbered four thousand nine hundred and fifty men, and lost in the assault eleven hundred men killed and wounded—six hundred and forty French and four hundred and sixty Americans.

This bloody repulse disheartened the besiegers, but General Lincoln still desired to continue the siege. In this he was opposed by Count d'Estaing, who feared to remain longer with his fleet, lest it should suffer from the autumnal gales. It was therefore determined to retreat. A bold front was shown the enemy while the ordnance and stores were being placed on the ships; and a

* The enemy buried their dead inside of the redoubt. In 1837 it was cut down to fill up a place where the Central Railroad depot now stands. A number of articles of warfare were dug up and are now in the possession of citizens.

few days after the assault the besiegers disappeared, the Americans retreated to Zubly's ferry, and the French re-embarked at Causton's bluff. The fleet sailed from Tybee on the 2d of November, encountering a heavy gale, which dispersed the ships.

Among the more noted personages killed and wounded during the assault were Counts d'Estaing and Pulaski, Major-General d'Fontagnes, Chevalier d'Ernonville, Colonel John White, Majors Pierce Butler and John Jones,* and Sergeant Jasper.

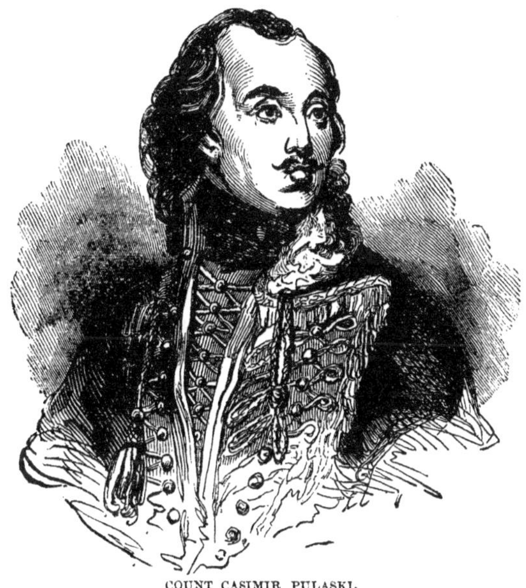

COUNT CASIMIR PULASKI.

Count Pulaski fell about the spot now occupied by the Central Railroad depot. He was born in the province of Lithuania, Poland, in the year 1746. He was elected leader of a band of patriots confederated together to relieve their native land from the oppressive rule of Russia. Austrian and Prussian troops were sent to assist the Russian forces stationed in Poland. Against these overwhelming odds the little band bravely contended, but was

* Instantly killed by a cannon-shot in front of the Spring Hill battery.

overpowered and the most severe punishments inflicted on those captured. Pulaski and other noblemen fled to France. Here he learned of the struggle of the Americans for independence, and tendered his services, which were accepted by Congress and the rank of Brigadier-General conferred upon him. Owing to the dissatisfaction of the officers under him he resigned, after having distinguished himself in several engagements. He was then empowered to raise a legion, which was soon after organized.

The Count, after his removal to the rear and the extraction of the ball from his groin, was placed on a vessel to be sent to Charleston. The vessel had hardly sailed out of the harbor before he died. The body immediately became so offensive that the captain was compelled to consign it to the depths of the sea.* The funeral services were performed in Charleston, where the announcement of the death of the brave Pole caused, as it did throughout the American colonies, the most intense grief.

Of Sergeant Jasper there is much of interest to relate. No braver and truer soldier died for the cause of American liberty. During the assault upon the Spring Hill redoubt he was conspicuous for his bravery and coolness. Though mortally wounded, he bore off the flag after vainly attempting to plant it inside of the redoubt. After the engagement Colonel Horry called to see him and found his life-blood ebbing fast. He was aware of his condition, and in a faint voice requested the Colonel to give the sword presented by Governor Rutledge to his father, and "tell him that I have worn it with honor, and if he should weep, tell him I died in the hope of a better life. Tell Mrs. Elliott I lost my life supporting the colors which she presented to our regiment. If you should ever see Jones, his wife, and son, tell them Jasper is gone, but that the remembrance of the battle† he fought for them brought a secret joy to his heart when it was about to stop its motion forever." He died a few moments after.

---

* There is great diversity of opinion in this regard, some asserting that he was buried at Greenwich, three miles from Savannah, and others on an island between here and Charleston. Captain Bentalou, an officer of Pulaski's staff, who was also wounded and on board of the vessel, wrote an account stating that Pulaski died on board and his body was thrown into the water because of its offensiveness, and in absence of other authority this must be accepted as correct.

† An account of the affair alluded to will be found under the head of Jasper Spring.

CHAPTER VI.

Appearance of the Town after the Siege — Riotous Negroes — Skirmishes around the Town — An American Dragoon Killed — He is scalped, stripped, his body dragged through the streets, and interment refused — Surrender of the Town by the British — Revival of Business — Organization of the Chatham Artillery — Burial of Major-General Greene — Shipment of the first Bale of Cotton — Incorporation of Savannah as a City — Visit of General Washington — His Account of his Visit and Description of the City — Destructive Fire in 1796 — Census of the City in 1798 — Visit of Vice-President Aaron Burr — Terrific Gale in 1804 — Savannah during the War of 1812 — Capture of the British Brig-of-war Epervier.

There were about four hundred houses in Savannah at the time of the siege * and about seven hundred and fifty inhabitants. A large number of the males were absent in the American army, and a great many families had fled the town to avoid the persecutions of the British. The batteries of the allies threw over a thousand shot and shell into the town, by which four houses were burned, several demolished, and a large number injured. The churches and public buildings had been used for hospitals and storehouses, and were not fit to be used for their original purposes. Governor Wright, who had made his appearance after the capture of the town in 1778, endeavored to restore it to its former condition; which he partially accomplished before its evacuation by the British forces. While the town was made an object of care and solicitude the inhabitants were not thought of, except as objects to impose fresh persecutions upon. Beside the petty tyrannies of the enemy the inhabitants had to bear the insolence of the negroes, who had first been employed by the enemy as laborers and then armed. This made them bold and overbearing; the females were insulted, and robbery and deeds of violence were committed. The people petitioned and petitioned Governor Wright to check the negroes; but his majesty allowed it to continue until it became so intolerable, not only to the citizens but to the British officers and soldiers also, that he was compelled to check them, and then found it a difficult matter.

* One hundred and sixty houses were so much injured by the soldiers and negroes, who had used them as quarters during the siege, as to be uninhabitable.

6*

Although the British were left in possession of the town they did not feel secure. They were kept constantly on the alert by small parties of Americans, who would dash up within view of their fortifications, capture all stragglers, pickets, and supplies, and be miles away before pursuit could be given. Among these detachments, the one under Captain John Bilbo * was the most noted. This petty warfare was continued near the town until early in 1782. Then General Wayne, with a small force of cavalry and artillery, was sent to the vicinity and operations were conducted on a larger scale, the enemy were kept close within the limits of the town, the provisions in the vicinity were destroyed, and when a sortie was made to interrupt the operations of the Americans the sallying party was made to suffer terribly. The British had some indians with them, and on one occasion an American dragoon was shot by them while charging with his troop near the batteries. General Wayne gives an account of the affair under date of the 20th of March, 1782, which says:

> When the enemy retreated they bore off the scalp of the dragoon, with which they paraded the streets of Savannah, headed by the Lieutenant-Governor and other British officers, who gave an entertainment to the indians and had a dance on the occasion. Nor did their barbarity rest here; they mangled and disfigured the dead body in a manner that none but wretches inured in acts of cruelty would possibly be capable of, and ordered it to remain unburied; but the Ethiopians, more humanized, stole it away and deposited it into the ground, for the commission of which crime a reward of five guineas is offered for the discovery of any person or persons concerned in that act of humanity.

On the 1st of July, 1782, General Wayne received, under a flag of truce, a deputation from the merchants of Savannah, who informed him that General Clarke, commandant of the town, daily expected orders to evacuate it, and they desired to ascertain upon what conditions the British subjects would be permitted to remain should that happen. General Wayne stated that he would give an answer the next day. He held a conference with Governor Martin, and when the deputation was presented he assured them that the persons and property of such as chose to remain in Savannah after it should be evacuated would be protected, and a reasonable

---

* Captain Bilbo's party, while attacking a party of the enemy a few miles from Savannah, was fired upon from a house, by which the captain was wounded. He was captured and brought to town, and died on the 8th of May, 1780. His death resulted from rough usage and neglect.

time would be allowed them to dispose of their property and settle their pecuniary affairs in the State, but that such men as had committed murder or other atrocious offences would be liable to be tried and punished according to the laws of the State. The deputation returned to town and communicated the reply to the inhabitants, who the next day appointed another deputation, with instructions to enter into definite terms and conditions and have them reduced to writing, which was accordingly done. Major John Habersham, a native of Savannah and an officer of the Georgia line, conducted the negotiations, which were satisfactory to both parties, especially to the British merchants, a number of whom decided to remain. The orders for the evacuation of the town came, and preparations were made to leave on the 11th of July and to surrender the town to the Americans the same day. By two o'clock on that day the British troops, twelve hundred in number, five hundred women and children, three hundred indians, five thousand negroes, and such other "plunder" as could be collected were on board of the vessels.* Two hours thereafter General Wayne issued the following order:

HEADQUARTERS, SAVANNAH, 11th July, 1782.

The light infantry company under Captain Parker to take post in the centre work in front of the town, placing sentinels at the respective gateways and sallyports, to prevent any person or persons going or entering the lines without written permits, until further orders.

No insults or depredations to be committed upon the persons or property of the inhabitants on any pretext whatever; the civil authorities only will take cognizance of the criminals or defaulters belonging to the State, if any there be.† The merchants and traders are immediately to take out an exact and true invoice of all goods; wares, and merchandise of every species, dry, wet, or hard, respectively belonging to them, or in their possession, with the original invoices, to the commissary, who will select such articles as may be necessary for the army and the public uses of the State, for which a reasonable profit will be allowed; no goods or merchandise of any kind whatsoever to be removed, secreted, sold, or disposed of until the public and army are first served; which will be as soon as possible after the receipt of the invoices, &c.

N. B. Orders will be left with Captain Parker for the immediate admission of the Honorable Executive Council and the Honorable members of the Legislature, with their officers and attendants.

A committee of British officers notified General Wayne that they

---

* The slaves were taken from the Georgia plantations.

† All of that class took care to get aboard of the British ships, and thus escaped the punishment they richly deserved.

were prepared to deliver up the keys, and formally surrendered the town. Colonel James Jackson, who had distinguished himself during the advance of the Americans and in the frequent skirmishes about the town, was selected by General Wayne to receive the surrender. That evening the American troops were paraded and marched to the principal gate, where the British officers stood with the keys. Colonel Jackson received them, and Savannah, which for three years six months and thirteen days had been under British rule, was free and in the possession of her own citizens. In the evening the British fleet sailed for England.

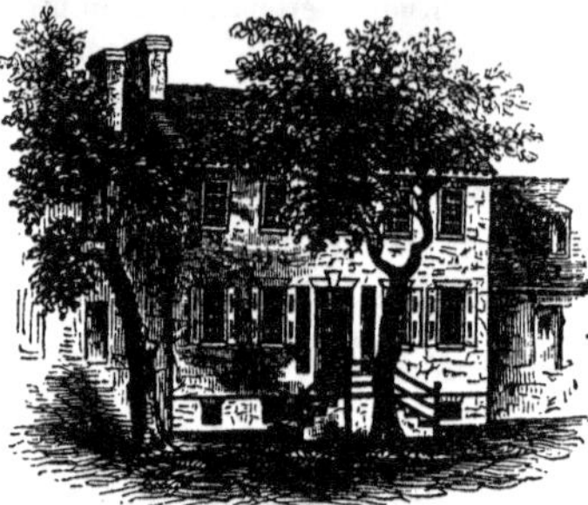
RESIDENCE OF GENERAL LACHLAN M'INTOSH.

Three weeks after, in pursuance of a call by Governor Martin for a special session, the State Legislature met in Savannah, in the house of General Lachlan McIntosh, situated on the north side of South Broad, third door east of Drayton street.

Soon after the evacuation all hostilities ceased between this and the mother country. The people went to work to repair the ravages of war. In Savannah the work was difficult—more so than elsewhere; the stringent rules of the British had prevented the citizens who remained in town from conducting business, and at the close of the war three fourths of the business houses were owned and controlled by others than natives of the town or of the United States—persons that were not trusted and who threw every obstacle in the way of all new business enterprises. Indomitable energy, at last, conquered; old firms were re-established, new ones organized, and a brisk trade was commenced with the neighboring ports. The public and private buildings were repaired, the streets and squares cleared of the *debris* of war, and the town assumed the beautiful and cleanly appearance it possessed in the "good old colony times."

On May 1st, 1786, the Chatham Artillery was organized, and on the 20th of June following was called upon to pay the soldier's tribute to the memory of Major-General Nathaniel Greene. This officer won undying fame in the Southern campaigns, and as a mark of appreciation of his services the Georgia Legislature granted him a large tract of land near Savannah. He settled upon this tract in 1783, and frequently visited town. On the 12th and 13th days of June, 1786, he was in Savannah and returned home on the 14th, on which day he was stricken down by an attack of *coup de soliel,* and died on the 19th. His remains were brought to Savannah the next day and interred with military honors in the old burying-ground on South Broad street. The procession, civic and military, was formed on the Bay and escorted the remains. The Chatham Artillery was in front firing minute-guns and advancing, and also fired a salute of thirteen guns at the grave.*

The first bale of cotton exported from Georgia was shipped from Savannah in 1788 by Thomas Miller. Mr. Miller was for a long time the only purchaser of cotton in Savannah. He bought it in parcels of from twenty-five to one hundred pounds, and assorted and packed it with his own hands. His exclusive and earnest attention to this branch of business earned for him the sobriquet, "Cotton" Miller.

Savannah was made a city by act of legislature in December, 1789, and the following year the first Mayor, John Houston, was elected.

May of the year after was made memorable by the visit of Washington to Savannah. The Georgia Gazette of the 19th devotes its entire space to an account of the visit, and says the President, with his committee, his Secretary, Majors Jackson and Butler, Gen. Wayne, and Mr. Baillie embarked at Purysburgh between ten and eleven o'clock on the 12th of May, and were rowed down the river by nine American captains, viz: Captains Putnam, Courtier, Rice, Fisher, Huntingdon, Kershaw, Swain, McIntire, and Morrison, who were dressed in light blue silk jackets, black satin breeches, white silk stockings, and round hats with black ribbons, bearing the words "LONG LIVE THE PRESIDENT" in letters of gold. Ten miles above the city the President and his escort were met by a large number of gentlemen in boats, and as the President passed by them a band played the celebrated song "He comes, the Hero comes," accompanied with several voices. On his approach to the city the "concourse on the bluff and the crowds which had pressed into the vessels evinced the general joy which had been inspired by the visit of this most beloved of men and the ardent desire of all ranks

---

* The vault in which the remains were placed was not designated at the time of interment. A search was made for them in 1820, but they could not be found.

and conditions of people to be gratified at his presence." He was received at the landing by General Jackson and Colonel Gunn, who introduced him to the Mayor and Aldermen. A procession was then formed and the guests were escorted to the quarters provided for them on St. James square. At six o'clock the President and suite dined at Brown's coffee-house, on the site now occupied by Stoddard's lower range, at which were present the Mayor of the city, President of the Cincinnati,* the Judges of the Superior courts of the State and Inferior courts of the county, clergy, members of the legislature, members of the Cincinnati, field officers of the militia, president of the Union society, and the Recorder and Treasurer of the city. The city was illuminated at night. Alderman Scheuber's house was brilliantly illuminated, "shewing no less than three hundred lights, arranged in a beautiful symmetry, with fifteen lights contained in the form of a W in front."

On the 13th the President partook of a dinner tendered by the Society of the Cincinnati. A ball was given in the long room of the filature at night. At half-past eight o'clock the President honored the company with his presence, and was personally introduced by one of the managers to ninety-six ladies, who were "elegantly dressed, some of whom displayed infinite taste in the emblems and devices on their sashes and head-dresses, out of respect to the happy occasion. After a few minuets were moved and one country dance led down, the President and his suite retired, about eleven o'clock. At two o'clock the supper-room was opened and the ladies partook of a repast, after which dancing continued until three o'clock."

On Saturday the President visited the old fortifications, and afterward partook of a dinner under an arbor with over two hundred citizens. The Chatham Artillery fired a gun between each toast offered, the last one of which, proposed by Washington, was "The present dexterous corps of artillery."† In the evening there was a handsome exhibition of fireworks, and "the amusements of this day of joy and festivity were crowned with a concert."

---

* The Cincinnati society was composed of officers of the American army.

† The President, soon after his visit, sent two brass six pounders as a present to the Chatham Artillery. These were used by the company until the late war. The frequent salutes fired by the battery rendered them unserviceable, and during the war they were buried. They will in time be exhumed and mingle their brazen voices upon occasions of joy which will mark the future history of Savannah.

On Sunday morning the President attended divine service in Christ church and soon after set out on his way to Augusta. On taking his leave of the Mayor and committee of the citizens he "politely expressed his sense of the attention shewn him by the corporation and every denomination of people during his stay in Savannah."

The account in the Gazette concludes with copies of the addresses presented to him and his replies to them. The committee, General Lachlan McIntosh, Colonels Noble Wimberly Jones and Joseph Habersham, and Messrs. John Houston and Joseph Clay, that met him at Purysburgh, T. H. Gibbons (Mayor), in behalf of himself and aldermen, George Houston, Masonic Grand Master of the State of Georgia, and General Anthony Wayne, president of the Cincinnati society, presented him with an address each. In reply to that of the committee, he concludes: "That the city of Savannah may largely partake of every public benefit which our free and equal government can dispense, and that the happiness of its vicinity may reply to the best wishes of its inhabitants, is my sincere prayer."

Washington kept a diary* during his trip. The following is his account *verbatim et literatem* of his reception in Savannah and his opinion of the city:

At that place (Purysburgh; 12th of May) I was met by Messrs Jones, Col. Habersham, Mr. John Houston, Genl. McIntosh and Mr. Clay, a comee. from the city of Savanna to conduct me thither. Boats were also ordered there by them for my accommodation, amon which a handsome 8 oared barge rowed by 8 American Captns. attended. In my way down the River I called upon Mrs. Green, the widow of the deceased Genl. Green (at a place called Mulberry Grove) & asked her how she did. At this place (2 miles from Purysburgh) my horses and Carriages were landed, and had 12 miles farther by Land to Savanna. The wind and tide being both agst. us, it was 6 o'clock before we reached the City, where were received under every demonstration that could be given of Joy & respect. We were Seven hours making the passage which is often performed in 4 tho the computed distance is 25 miles—Illums. at night.

I was conducted by the Mayor & Wardens to very good lodging which had been provided for the occasion, and partook of a public dinner given by the Citizens at the Coffee Room. At Purisburgh I parted with Gen. Moultree.

Friday, 13th—Dined with the Members of the Cincinnati at a public dinner given at the same place—and in the evening went to a dancing Assembly at which there was about 100 well dressed & handsome ladies.

Saturday 14th. A little after 6 o'clock, in Company with Genl. McIntosh, Genl

* Mr. Benson J. Lossing has recently published his diaries in book form, entitled "Washington's Private Diaries," from which this account is taken.

Wayne, the Mayor, and many others (principal Gentlemen of the City) I visited the City, and the attack and defence of it in the year 1779, under the combined forces of France and the United States, commanded by Count de Estaing & Gen. Lincoln.—To form an opinion of the attack at this distance of time, and the change which has taken place in the appearance of the ground by the cutting away of the woods, &c. is hardly to be done with Justice to the subject; especially as there is remaining scarcely any of the defences.

Dined to day with a number of the Citizens (not less than 200) in an elegant bower erected for the occasion on the Bank of the River below the Town. In the evening there was a tolerable good display of fireworks.

Sunday 15th—After morning service, and receiving a number of visits from the most respectable ladies of the place (as was the case yesterday) I set out for Augusta, Escorted beyd. the limits of the City by most of the Gentlemen in it, and dining at Mulberry Grove the seat of Mrs. Green—lodged at one Spencers—distant 15 miles.

Savanna stands upon what may be called high ground for this Country—It is extremely sandy wch. makes the walking very disagreeable; and the houses very uncomfortable in warm and windy weather, as they are filled with dust whenever these happen. The Town on 3 sides is surrounded with cultivated Rice fields which have a rich and luxuriant appearance. On the 4th or backside it is a fine sand. The harbour is said to be very good & often filled with square rigged vessels, but there is a bar below over which not more than 12 water can be brot. except at sprg tides. The tide does not flow above 12 or 14 miles above the City though the river is swelled by it more than double that distance. Rice and Tobacco (the last of wch. is greatly increasing) are the principal Exports. Lumber and Indigo are also Exported, but the latter is on the decline, and it is supposed by Hemp and Cotton.—Ship timber. viz: live oak & cedar, is (and may be more so) valuable in the exptn.

At the time of Washington's visit there were no houses beyond South Broad street, and only five upon that street, all being on the north side. The city limits on the east was Lincoln street, and on the west Jefferson street, although there were a number of houses west of the latter-named street. Of the five houses then standing on South Broad street four remain, viz: "Eppinger's house,"* on the northeast corner of Jefferson street, now occupied by Mr. S. Davis; the old frame house between Barnard and Jefferson; the frame house at the northeast corner of Whitaker; and the old brick house the third door east of Drayton street, now occupied by

---

* There is a record showing that Eppinger built this house previous to the year 1747. He used it as a public house, and at his death his son occupied it as a residence, and opened a public house in the old brick house on South Broad street—the oldest brick house in Savannah. The room in which the State legislature met previous to the removal of the capitol of the State to Augusta was known as "Eppinger's Long Room," in which balls and public meetings were held during the week and religious services on Sunday.

Mr. John B. Robinson; the fifth house stood where a brick house has just been completed, between Drayton and Abercorn streets.

The fine and flourishing prospects of this rapidly growing commercial city, which had just fully emerged from the ruinous effects of the late war, were totally suspended by a destructive fire on the 26th of November, 1796, which destroyed two hundred and twenty-nine buildings, exclusive of out-houses, causing a loss of more than a million of dollars. It broke out in a bake-shop near the market and swept in every direction—some families having to move their furniture seven different times to avoid the flames. Hundreds of families were rendered houseless and hundreds thrown out of employment. The suffering and distress was great, notwithstanding the generous donations of money and provisions from all parts of the State. The people, with that energy which has ever characterized them, strove to retrieve their losses, meeting with that success which always attends well-directed exertion.

A census of the city was taken in 1798, and it was ascertained that there were 6,226 inhabitants, 237 of them negroes; 618 dwelling-houses, 415 kitchens, 228 out-houses, stores, and shops.

Vice-President Aaron Burr visited the city on the 20th of May, 1802, coming from Augusta. As he approached he was saluted by the Chatham Artillery, posted on Spring hill, and was escorted into Savannah by the Chatham Rangers and Savannah Volunteer Guards. He remained three or four days; but very little attention was paid him—no more than the formal ceremonies his position called for. The paper of that day (the Georgia Gazette) devotes only fifteen lines to an account of the visit, and does not mention his name.

On the 8th of September, 1804, a storm raged with destructive fury from 9 A. M. to 10 P. M. None of the inhabitants dared to venture out, excepting those who had to flee to avoid being crushed in the ruins of their own houses. The river rose above the wharves, and covered Hutchinson's island and the rice-plantations around the city. The Gazette says the people who had been kept in the house the day before, their fancies depicting a most woeful scene, found, the next morning, that busy fancy, ever prone to exaggerate, had formed but an imperfect picture of the dreadful scene of havoc and destruction. A large number of trees in every part of the city were blown down, and also several houses, the steeple of the Presbyterian meeting-house, and part of the walls of the Episcopal (Christ) church. The wharves from one end of the city to the other were torn up, and many storehouses erected at the foot of the bluff were either totally destroyed or so much torn to pieces as to render valueless everything within them. Every vessel in the harbor was thrown upon the wharves, except such as were totally destroyed. In the city several persons were injured by falling houses and chimneys, and two of Mr. Green's children were instantly killed. Captain Webb was also killed. Twenty-four houses, including the exchange, the filature, jail, and court-house on the bluff, and twenty-six business houses under the bluff, were injured and their stocks of goods swept away. Eighteen vessels were swept upon the wharves and there remained when the water subsided. Over one hundred negroes were drowned on Hutchinson's island and on the rice-plantations near the city. The steeple of the Presbyterian church (then situated where now stands the large brick livery stables on the southwest corner of Whitaker and President streets) which was nearly as high as the present steeple of the Independent Presbyterian church, fell in a southwesterly direction, crushing in a house and cutting off a portion of a bed on which lay a sick man, fortunately not injuring him. The bell in the steeple was found, much to the astonishment of all, unbroken. It was afterward hung in the steeple of the Independent Presbyterian church, and there remained until about 1824, when a larger bell was presented to the congregation.

During the war of 1812, between the United States and England, Savannah was not attacked, but its proximity to the sea made it liable to assault by the enemy's fleets at almost any hour, and thus the people were kept constantly upon the alert until peace was restored in 1815. Fort Wayne was still fortified. Another fort was erected about two and a half miles below the city and named Fort Jackson, after Governor James Jackson. A line of defences was thrown up, extending from the marsh on the east at the foot of Broughton street to the west side of Lafayette square, where the residence of Andrew Low now stands, thence diverging to what is now Liberty Street lane, thence crossing Bull street to Spring hill, where the Central Railroad depot is now, thence along the high ground east of the Ogeechee canal, and terminating at what is now the foot of Farm street. The line was very irregular and unusually full of salients and re-entering angles. The old volunteer companies,* Chatham Artillery, Savannah Volunteer

* These companies, with all others of the Confederate army, were disbanded by order of the United States, in 1865, having participated in the war between the Southern and Northern States.

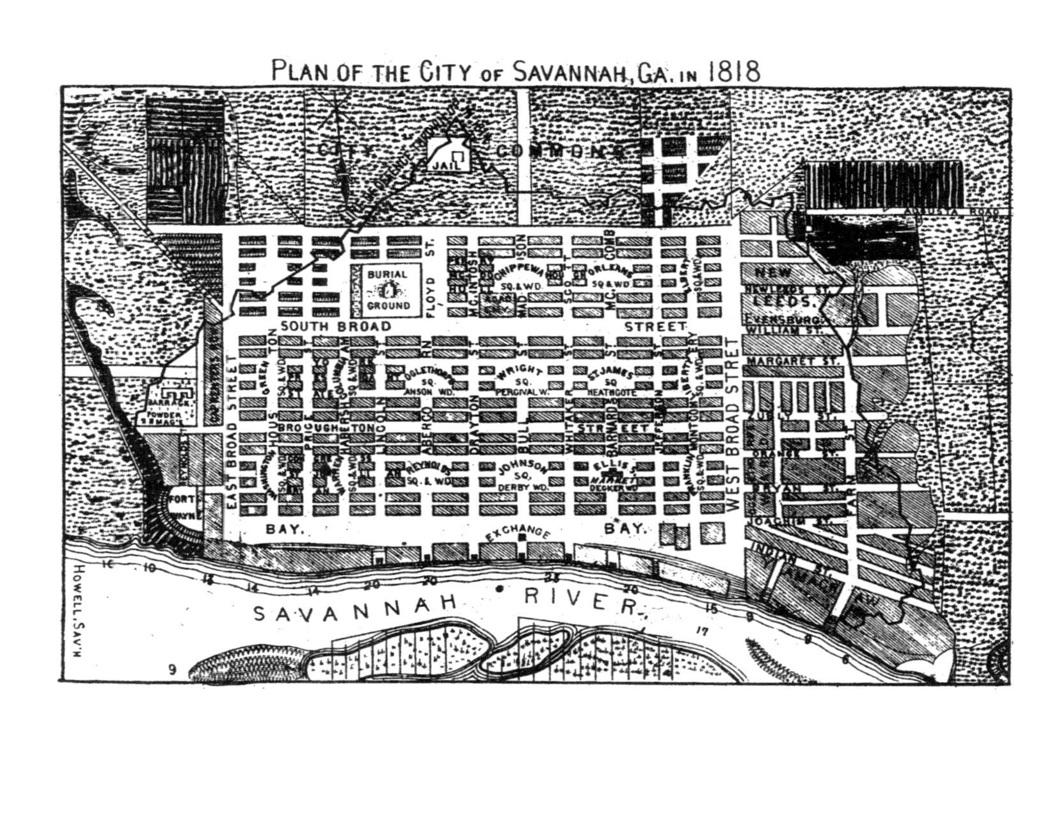

PLAN OF THE CITY OF SAVANNAH, GA. IN 1818

Guards, Republican Blues, and Georgia Hussars, and other companies which organized for the war, and of which no record can be found, were constantly on duty. Early in the war half of the members of the Savannah Volunteer Guards and the Republican Blues were sent on an expedition against St. Augustine, Florida; but before arrangements for the assault were made, Florida was purchased by the United States. The only surviving member of the two Savannah companies that participated in this expedition is Mr. Jacob Miller. He and Mr. O. M. Lillibridge are the only living representatives of this city in that war. Both were members of the Republican Blues; the former is seventy-nine and the latter eighty-two years of age.

In May, 1814, the Epervier, a British brig-of-war, built in 1812, carrying eighteen guns, was brought into the river by the United States sloop-of-war Peacock, Lewis Warrington commander. The Epervier had on board, when captured, one hundred and ten thousand dollars in specie, which were confiscated and distributed according to law.

CHAPTER VII.

Arrival of the Steamship Savannah — Visit of President Monroe — Terrible Conflagration in 1820 — Yellow Fever in the same Year — Visit of General Lafayette — Departure of the Irish Jasper Greens for Mexico — Visit of President Filmore — Yellow Fever in 1854 — Terrible Gale the same Year — The Secession Movement — Hoisting of the Secession Flag — Election of Delegates to the State Convention — Seizure of Fort Pulaski, Fort Jackson, and Oglethorpe Barracks — Reassembling of the State Convention — Saluting the Flag of the Confederate States — Departure of the Oglethorpe Light Infantry for Virginia — Burial of General Bartow—Placing Obstructions in the river — Arrival of General Robert E. Lee — Reduction of Fort Pulaski — Threatening Demonstrations of the Enemy—Resolution of Council to Defend the City to the last Extremity — General Lawton Ordered to Virginia, and General Mercer placed in command of Savannah — Capture of the iron-clad Atlanta by the Federals, and capture of the armed steamer Water Witch by the Confederates — Arrival of General Sherman's army in front of Savannah — Storming of Fort McAlister — Evacuation of Savannah by the Confederate Forces—Its Surrender by Members of the Council—Entrance of the Federal Troops — General Sherman's Order — Meeting of the Citizens—A surprise for a "Blockader"—Drowning of Federal Soldiers on Hutchinson's Island — Intrenchments thrown up by the Federals — Destructive Fire and Novel Bombardment — The Wives and Children of Officers of the Confederate Army and Navy sent out of the City.

The first steamship ever built in the United States was projected and owned in this city. It was built North and named Savannah. In April, 1819, it arrived here from New York, and in a few days after sailed for Liverpool, accomplishing the voyage in twenty-two days, the sails being used only eight days. Vessels propelled by steam were a rarity in those days, and the idea of steam being used in connection with sails, and a vessel of that description crossing the ocean, had never been thought of in Great Britain. When the Savannah arrived off Cape Clear she was signalled to Liverpool as a vessel on fire, and a cutter was sent from Cork to her relief. Great was the "surprise and admiration when she entered the harbor of Liverpool under bare poles, belching forth smoke and fire, yet uninjured." The return voyage occupied twenty-five days.

James Monroe, the fifth President of the United States, visited Savannah in May, 1819, and was received with that hospitality for which Savannah has always been noted.

On the 11th of January, 1820, after a lapse of twenty-four years, Savannah again experienced the horrors of a conflagration, far surpassing in violence and destruction that of 1796. The fire broke out about two o'clock A. M. in the livery stable of Mr. Boon, situated near the market. The wind was high, and before the flames were extinguished four hundred and sixty-three houses, exclusive of out-buildings, were destroyed. With the exception of the State and Planter's banks, the Episcopal church, and three or four other brick buildings, every house between Broughton and Bay streets, from Jefferson to Abercorn streets, were destroyed. The loss was estimated at four million dollars.

The people had barely recovered from the shock caused by this great disaster and commenced to rebuild before pestilence interrupted the work and swept many into their graves. On the 5th of September a vessel arrived from the West Indies, having the yellow fever on board. A day or two after, several cases were reported in the city. It spread quite rapidly, and before it was checked, on the 6th of November following, two hundred and thirty-nine persons had been stricken down by it. The number of inhabitants at the time it commenced was 7,523. The dread of the fever caused many to flee from the city. A census was taken late in October, when it was ascertained that there were only 1,494 persons remaining in the city, and that three hundred and forty-three houses were uninhabited. The loss of life was mostly confined to the foreign population who had come the winter previous.

General Lafayette arrived in Savannah from Charleston on the 18th of March, 1825. His arrival was made the occasion of one of the largest and most imposing civic and military displays ever before witnessed in Savannah. He landed at the east end of the bluff, and was received with the usual salutes and ceremonies. At seven o'clock a dinner was served in the Exchange. In the centre window, in the rear of General Lafayette and the Mayor, appeared a transparency of General Lafayette, over which was a scroll inscribed "He Fought for Us." In the opposite window was a transparency of Washington, with the inscription "The Father of his Country." The centre window in front presented an allegorical transparency, representing a monument surmounted with a bust of Lafayette—on one side Liberty, on the other History presenting a tablet inscribed with the dates of the general's arrival in America, his appointment as Major-General, his being wounded at Brandywine, and of the surrender at Yorktown. During the general's stay in Savannah the corner-stone of the monument to General Greene was laid in Johnson square, and one for a monument to General Pulaski in Chippewa square, with the most imposing ceremonies.

In the year 1846 hostilities between the United States and Mexico commenced, and a call was made upon Georgia for a regiment of soldiers, to be sent to the seat of war. The regiment was promptly raised and sent off under Colonel Henry R. Jackson, and shared the honors won by our soldiers on the Mexican plains. The Irish Jasper Greens, of Savannah, were with the regiment, the following named officers and men composing the company: J. McMahon, Captain; G. Curlette, D. O'Connor, Lieutenants; John Devaney, M. Carey, P. Martin, Sergeants; Leo Wylly, M. Feery, P. Tierney, T. Bourke, Owen Reilly, Corporals; William Bandy, W. D. Burke, P. Bossu, Francis Camfield, J. Chalmers, P. Clark, P. Cody, John Coffee, William Coffee, James Conlihan, Elijah Condon, Joseph Davis, Dennis Dermond, Michael Downy, Michael Duggan, Francis Dutzmer, Charles Farrelly, Thomas Fenton, David Fountain, James Fleeting, James Flynn, William P. Fielding, James Feely, P. Gerrin, Moses Gleason, O. B. Hall, Michael Hoar, Timothy Howard, R. M. Howard, E. W. Irwin, John Keegin, Humphrey Leary, W. S. Levi, David Lynch, Michael Lynch, L. Mahoney, Henry Marry, John Makin, Bryan Morris, James McFehilly, Hugh Murtagh, Henry Nagle, Daniel Nickels, M. M. Payne, George Perminger, Thomas Pigeon, John Reagan, Francis Reeves, R. Richardson, J. Rinehart, B. Rodebuck, R. M. Robertson, J. D. Ryan, Thomas Ryan, John Sanderlyn, Michael Shea, Peter Suzmel, David Stokes, C. F. E. Smyth, R. L. S. Smith, Patrick Shiels, Patrick Tidings, Daniel F. Fowles, J. W. Warden, James Waters, Michael Weldon, John Whaling, James Waters, jr., Jacob Zimmerman, privates; William Gatehouse, George Gatehouse, musicians.

On the 22d of April, 1854, President Filmore, accompanied by the Hon. J. P. Kennedy, arrived in Savannah per Central railroad and was received by a large concourse of citizens, the Chatham Artillery firing a salute as the train came in. Quarters were provided for the guests at the Pulaski House. A ball was given at St. Andrews Hall, a trip made to Fort Pulaski, and everything that could contribute to the pleasure and comfort of the distinguished guests was cheerfully done during their stay.

On the 12th of August, 1854, yellow fever made its appearance among the residents of Washington ward. In a short time it spread through the city, the mortality reaching its maximum height about the 12th of September, on which day fifty-one interments were reported. The decline of the sickness commenced about the 20th of September, and on the 29th of October only one interment was reported. The last death by the fever occurred on the 29th of November. Two thirds of the permanent white population left the city when the fever commenced to spread, leaving six thousand persons to brave the disease—a large mrjority of whom were sick.

On the 8th of September, and during the prevalence of the fever, a severe and destructive storm visited Savannah. Hutchinson and Fig islands were covered with water, and a number of houses washed away and persons drowned. The light-house on the latter island was washed away. The timber in Willink's ship-yard was floated off and the yard injured. Baldwin's cotton-press and the buildings at A. N. Miller's foundry were unroofed. Nearly all of the trees on South Broad street were blown down. Most of the shipping in the river was driven upon the wharves and sustained considerable damage. The large dry-dock parted from her moorings and floated up the river, but was secured after running afoul of and damaging several vessels. The loss sustained was never fully ascertained, but was very heavy,

Never in the history of Savannah had the hand of affliction fallen so heavily upon her as during this epidemic season, when disease wasted the lives and paralyzed the energies of her citizens, and the tempest and tides threatened to complete the general destruction. During these calamities the active sympathy of the benevolent everywhere was enlisted, and contributions of money and provisions poured in from every quarter. Those who extended aid will long be held in grateful remembrance by the people of Savannah, who, when in the dispensation of Providence other communities may be overtaken by misfortune, will be as prompt to extend aid as they were thankful to receive it.

The Secession movement of the Southern States in 1860 met the hearty approval of the citizens of Savannah, which was the first city in the State to move in the glorious cause of resistance to Radical rule. The announcement of the secession of South Carolina, in December of this year, was hailed with delight and created the wildest enthusiasm. A secession flag, bearing the representation of a large rattlesnake, with the inscription "DON'T TREAD ON ME," was unfurled from the top of the Greene monument, in Johnson square. Patriotic speeches were made, and every assurance given that the citizens would heartily co-operate with South Carolina. The old volunteer companies, the Chatham Artillery, Savannah Volunteer Guards, Republican Blues, Georgia Hussars, Phœnix Riflemen, Irish Jasper Greens, Oglethorpe Light Infantry, DeKalb Riflemen, and German Volunteers, promptly tendered their services for any duty that might be required of them. Their ranks were daily increased by volunteers and numerous other companies were organized.

The call for a State convention to assemble at once and act upon the question of secession originated in Savannah, and met with ready response throughout the State. On the 2d of January, 1861, an election for delegates to the convention was held. Captain Francis S. Bartow, Captain John W. Anderson, and Colonel A. S. Jones, nominees of the party favoring immediate secession and separate State action, were unanimously elected.

The citizens of Savannah, after hearing of the evacuation of Fort Moultrie and occupation of Fort Sumter by the United States forces under Major Anderson, determined to seize Fort Pulaski, being convinced that the policy of the United States government was to provoke a war, and in furtherance of the policy would hold all the forts commanding the harbors of the Southern States. A meeting of the citizens was held in a room in Battersby's buildings, at the southwest corner of Bay and Drayton streets, at which were present all of the officers and a number of men of the volunteer companies of Savannah. It was determined to seize and occupy the fort whether sanctioned by the Governor or not, but as a matter of prudence he was notified and his permission asked, which was granted. Accordingly, on the third day of January, 1861, Colonel A. R. Lawton marshalled the Savannah Volunteer Guards, Captain (now Colonel) John Screven; the Oglethorpe Light Infantry, Captain Francis S. Bartow (afterward promoted to the rank of Brigadier-General, and killed at the battle of Manassas), and two detachments from the Chatham Artillery, Captain (now Colonel) Joseph S. Claghorn, and proceeded to the fort and took formal possession of it in the name of the State of Georgia—the small garrison, under command of an ordnance sergeant, making no resistance.

The adoption of the ordinance of secession by the State convention at Milledgeville was hailed with a delight equal to that manifested at the secession of South Carolina. All prepared for the conflict which they saw was inevitable. General A. R. Lawton was placed in command of this department, and under his orders Fort Jackson and the Oglethorpe barracks were seized and occupied by Savannah's soldiers.

The State convention reassembled in Savannah, in the Masonic hall, on the seventh day of March, 1861, and after framing a constitution for the State adjourned on the 23d of March.

The day after the assembling of the convention the flag of the Confederate States of America was thrown to the breeze from the Custom House staff by Major W. J. McIntosh. A salute of seven guns—one for each State of the Confederacy—was fired in honor of the occasion.

The Oglethorpe Light Infantry, Captain Francis S. Bartow, requested, but did not receive permission,* to go to Virginia, and departed without it on the 21st of May, being escorted to the cars by the volunteer companies of the city and a large concourse of citizens, who wished the company God speed, little dreaming that in a few short weeks they would, while rejoicing over a great victory, be also mourning the loss of its late gallant captain and a number of its no less gallant members. But so was it to be. The telegraph, on the 22d of July, 1861, brought the news of the great victory at Manassas, at the same time telling of the deaths of General Francis S. Bartow and a number of his old command, who had fallen in the thickest of the fray.

The remains of Bartow were brought from the field and forwarded to this city via Charleston, at which place, in honor to his memory, the public buildings were draped in mourning and the remains escorted through the city by the military and the citizens, the whole community vieing with one another in showing respect to the fallen brave. The remains arrived in the night of the 27th of July, and were escorted from the depot to the Exchange by the Oglethorpe Light Infantry (company B) and detachments from the other city companies, all under command of Captain F. W. Sims, the Chatham Artillery firing minute-guns as the escort moved. On the 28th the funeral of the deceased took place, and was the most solemn and imposing spectacle ever witnessed in Savannah. At three o'clock P. M. the military escort, consisting of all the city companies and detachments from the troops stationed in

* General Bartow's communication regarding the refusal of Governor Brown to allow his company to go to Virginia, will be found with the biographical sketch of the general.

the vicinity, formed on the Bay and escorted the remains to Christ church, which was thronged in every part with citizens. The funeral services were conducted by Right Reverend Stephen Elliott, Bishop of Georgia; after which the remains were carried to Laurel Grove cemetery, where with military honors they were consigned to their final resting place. The universal expression of sadness was truly impressive, and proved how sincerely the entire community deplored the loss of one who was not less loved in life than honored in his glorious death.

The bombardment and capture of Port Royal in November of 1861 occasioned intense excitement in Savannah, as it was believed that the large Federal fleet employed there would next attack the city. While all were sensible of the danger that threatened Savannah, yet they did not despair of being able to successfully combat it. The paving-stones on the Bay and along the slips were torn up and placed on board of vessels, which were towed down the river and sunk across the channel, and batteries were erected to command the obstructions. All that could be accomplished was done by General Lawton and the officers and men under his command.

General Robert E. Lee, then commander-in-chief of the Southern coast defences, arrived in Savannah on the 11th of November, and remained until the February following. He visited all of the fortifications and approved of the measures adopted for the defence of the city. He examined Fort Pulaski and expressed the opinion that its walls would withstand the heaviest cannon.*

A portion of the enemy's fleet appeared off Tybee shortly after the bombardment of Port Royal, but made no general demonstration, the commander apparently contenting himself by shelling our batteries and replying to the compliments sent now and then from Commodore Tatnall's little fleet, yet really preparing for the reduction of Fort Pulaski. This fort, the siege and reduction of which will ever be a memorable event in the history of the late war, is situated on Cockspur island, fourteen miles from the city, and was named after Brigadier-General Count Pulaski. The site of the fort was selected by Major Babcock, United States corps of engineers, and the work commenced in 1831, under the superintendence of Captain (now Major-General) Mansfield, United States army. The work was erected to command both channels of the Savannah

* Rifled cannon of large calibre had not been tested then, and their penetrative power was of course unknown.

river at the head of the Tybee roads. It was sixteen years in building, and its massive walls contained over thirteen million bricks, and cost about a million of dollars. It has five faces, including the gorge, and casemated on all sides. The walls are seven and a half feet thick, rising twenty-five feet above the water. The fort called for an armament of one hundred and forty guns, one tier in embrasure and one *en barbette*. The gorge is covered by an earthwork—it and the main work being surrounded and divided by a wide wet-ditch.

As has been stated, the work was taken possession of on the 3d of January, 1861. The captors found that only twenty thirty-two pounders were mounted; that there were no ordnance nor other stores, and everything generally out of order. But with that spirit which ever characterized the troops of Georgia the new garrison went to work, and in a short time placed the fort on a war-footing, having mounted forty-eight serviceable guns, the heaviest being ten-inch columbiads. When the Federals seized and commenced to fortify Tybee island early in 1862, the fort was considered impregnable to an assault, and as the power of rifled ordnance was then unknown, no one ever dreamed that its walls could be breached. The Federals, under cover of their gunboats, worked day and night erecting batteries. The garrison was also employed in strengthening the defences of the fort. On the 22d of February, 1862, the enemy succeeded in passing their vessels through Wall's cut and entered the Savannah river above the fort, thus cutting it off from all communication with Savannah. Just previous to this Commodore Tatnall managed with his little fleet, notwithstanding the formidable resistance made by the Federal gunboats, to effect a passage of the Savannah river, and threw into the fort a six months' supply of provisions. By the 10th of April the Federals had erected eleven sand batteries upon Tybee island. These batteries, distributed along a front of two thousand five hundred and fifty yards, mounted thirty-six heavy guns—ten heavy rifled cannon among them—and a number of mortars. These guns were well protected. The farthest was three thousand four hundred, and the nearest one thousand six hundred and fifty yards from the fort. Early on the morning of the tenth General David Hunter, commanding the besieging force, sent, under a flag of truce, an order "for the immediate surrender and restoration of Fort Pulaski to the authority and possession of the United States," to which Colonel Charles H. Olmstead, commandant of the fort, after acknowledging the receipt of the order, heroically and laconically replied: "I am here to defend the fort, not to surrender it." A few minutes after the return of the flag of truce the enemy opened on the fort from battery Halleck, followed by the other batteries, viz: Stanton, Grant, Lyon, Lincoln, Burnside, Sherman, Scott, Sigel, McClellan, and Totten. They continued firing until dark. The fort replied slowly, the gunners having to aim at the puffs of smoke, there being nothing else to indicate the position of the hostile guns. At eleven o'clock at night the firing was resumed by the enemy, and in the morning it became general. At midday all but two of the casemate guns bearing upon Tybee were dismounted, and but two of the barbette guns that could bear upon the batteries doing the most damage were left; the outer walls of two of the casemates were shot away, and two adjoining ones were in a crumbling condition; the moat was bridged over by the ruins of the walls; most of the traverses were riddled, and some of them no longer serviceable, the range of officers' quarters and kitchens was badly damaged, and the north magazine in hourly danger of explosion. The communications were so completely cut off that there was no ground for even the shadow of a hope of relief, and for the same reason no line of retreat was left. Under these circumstances Colonel Olmstead rightly considered the fort untenable, and, believing the lives of his command to be his next care, gave the necessary orders for a surrender, having first conferred with his officers and found them like himself thoroughly impressed with the conviction of the utter hopelessness of a longer struggle. The garrison then numbered about three hundred and sixty-five men and twenty-five officers, composed of the following companies: German Volunteers, Captain John H. Stegin; Washington Volunteers, Captain John McMahon; Wise Guards, Captain M. J. McMullen; Oglethorpe Light Infantry (company B), Captain F. W. Sims; Montgomery Guards, Captain L. J. Guilmartin. The field and staff officers were: Colonel Charles H. Olmstead, Commandant of Post; Major John Foley; W. H. Hopkins, Adjutant; Robert Erwin, Quartermaster; Robert D. Walker, Commissary; T. J. McFarland, Surgeon; Robert H. Lewis, Sergeant-Major; W. C. Crawford, Quartermaster's Sergeant; Harvey Lewis, Ordnance Sergeant; Edward D. Hopkins, Quartermaster's Clerk; E. W. Drummond, Commissary's Clerk.

The members of the garrison were sent to Hilton Head and then to New York, where they were confined until a general exchange was effected. Their conduct during the trying days of the siege, bombardment, and imprisonment was most heroic, and Savannah, of which nearly all are natives, is justly proud of them and their deeds. Only eighteen members of the garrison were wounded—four seriously, the others slightly—although three thousand shot and shell were thrown into the fort. The Federals admitted a loss of several killed and wounded and considerable damage to their guns and works.

On the second day, when the enemy's fire was hottest, the halyards of the flag of the fort were cut away and the flag fell. Lieutenant Christopher Hussey,* of the Montgomery Guards, and John Latham, of the Washington Volunteers, immediately sprang upon the parapet, and seizing the flag carried it to a gun-carriage at the northeastern angle of the fort, where they rigged a temporary staff, from which the flag proudly floated until the surrender.

Reverend Father P. Whelan was in the fort during the siege, and by his calmness and cheering words did much to encourage the members of the garrison during their severe ordeal. After the surrender he was offered his liberty, but refused to accept the offer, and underwent all the rigors of imprisonment with those he loved and to whom he was endeared. This noble old christian hero, after his release, administered to the wants of the sick and wounded in many localities. He is now in Savannah attending to his clerical duties as far as his feeble health will permit. May his days be long on the earth is the earnest prayer of hundreds of soldiers throughout the United States, and especially the Catholics of this city and elsewhere.

Since the war the fort has been considerably repaired, yet there still remain thousands of marks which speak of the terrible power of rifled guns. Travelers going out and coming into the Savannah river can readily observe the battered condition of the walls of Fort Pulaski, and now and then catch a glimpse of the sand batteries, behind which the enemy worked the guns which told so fearfully upon the fort.

The reduction of Fort Pulaski and the subsequent movements of the Federals confirmed the opinion that Savannah was to be attacked, but the result has shown that they were only feints, intended to distract the attention of our authorities and keep a

* Lieutenant Hussey died a few days before General Joseph E. Johnston's surrender, from the effects of rigorous imprisonment.

large force here while they prosecuted hostile operations elsewhere. The military authorities being convinced that the city would be attacked, determined to defend it to the last extremity, which determination met the cordial approval of the citizens, as also did the adoption of the following preamble and resolutions, offered by Alderman Hiram Roberts at a special meeting of the City Council held on the 29th of April, 1862:

WHEREAS, A communication has been received from the commanding General, stating that he will defend this city to the last extremity, and whereas, the members of the Council unanimously approve of the determination of the commanding General, therefore be it

Resolved, That the Council will render all the aid that is in their power to sustain the General and to carry out his laudable determination.

In May, 1862, General Lawton was ordered to report to General Lee in Virginia with five thousand men, and departed shortly after the reception of the order. His brigade participated in the many battles fought by the grand old army of northern Virginia and was greatly distinguished for its gallant conduct. After the departure of General Lawton General Hugh W. Mercer was placed in command of this district, and thus remained until Lieutenant-General W. J. Hardee assumed command in 1864, a short time prior to the evacuation of the city.

About July, 1863, the ironclad ship Atlanta, on which every effort and all means at command had been used to render her a forminable vessel, steamed down to Warsaw sound to attack the ironclad monitors Weehawken and Nahant, which were awaiting her coming. When within a few hundred yards of them she ran aground, but was immediately backed off, only to run more firmly aground again while sailing toward her opponents. While in this unfortunate condition, unable to extricate herself or bring her guns to bear, the ironclads opened upon her with fifteen-inch guns at short range. The fire was very effective, and in sixteen minutes after its commencement the iron armor and wood backing of the Atlanta had been seriously damaged and sixteen men wounded—among them, two out of the three pilots. Under these circumstances her commander, Captain Webb, wisely concluded to surrender. The Atlanta was armed with four superior rifled guns and manned with a fine crew and efficient officers. Her capture was greatly deplored, as she had been relied upon to protect the harbor from the enemy's ironclads, and her loss left the harbor almost unprotected, excepting by obstructions and land batteries. The

Atlanta was formerly the Fingal, which, under the command of Captain Edward C. Anderson, the present Mayor of the city, had been run through the blockade of the river early in the war, laden with munitions of war and other valuable goods, which were much needed by the government.

An offset to the capture of the Atlanta was the boarding and capture of the Water Witch by Lieutenant Pelot on the night of the second of June, 1864. The Water Witch formed one of the blockading squadron of the coast of Georgia, and was lying in Ossabaw sound. Lieutenant Pelot, with eighty men, embarked in seven barges and arrived near the Water Witch about half-past one o'clock. A dash for the steamer was immediately made, and after fifteen minutes hand-to-hand conflict (during which, and almost at the moment of victory, Lieutenant Pelot fell, pierced to the heart with a bullet) the crew surrendered. The Confederates lost six killed and twelve wounded. The enemy's crew, eighty-two in number, lost two killed and fifteen wounded, the commander, Lieutenant Prendergast, being among the latter. The capture of the steamer, armed with four heavy guns, eighty prisoners, and her equipment entire, was the result of this bold enterprise.

Nothing out of the usual line of petty skirmishes, reconnoissances, and the like, occurred around Savannah until the 11th of December, 1864, when Sherman's army arrived in front of the line of defences, his force amounting to sixty thousand infantry, six thousand cavalry, and a full supply of artillery. Along the coast was a large fleet of ironclads and other war vessels, awaiting the establishment of communication with the enemy's land force, to co-operate with it in the siege of the city. To oppose this force Lieutenant-General William J. Hardee had ten thousand men of all arms.

The movements of the enemy were closely watched by General Hardee, and everything that human foresight could devise to embarrass and repel their advance was accomplished; in which efforts he was sustained by Generals Hugh W. Mercer, Henry R. Jackson, W. R. Boggs, J. F. Gilmer, George P. Harrison, Colonel J. G. Clarke, and all of the officers and men under their command. The citizens volunteered their services, and stood in the trenches ready and willing to risk their lives in defence of their loved and beautiful city from the hands of the marauders, whose conduct during their "march to the sea" would have disgraced savages.

The enemy's first object was to establish communication with the fleet and obtain provisions, of which they stood in sore need.

Fort McAllister, which was so ably defended in numerous instances by the soldiers of Savannah, constituted the right of the outer line of the defences of the city, and was situated on Genesis Point, on the right bank of the Great Ogeechee river, and was intended to dispute a passage up the river and to prevent depredations in that vicinity. This fort, a strong earthwork, was the only barrier in the way of establishing the desired communication, and its capture was determined upon by Sherman. Before relating the account of its capture it would not be amiss to take a retrospective glance and give a brief history of this work, the defence of which reflected the utmost credit upon the garrison, and will send its name down to history with those of Arcola, Malakoff, and Donelson. It is situated about sixteen miles from Savannah, and was among the first of the numerous earthworks constructed for the defence of the city, but was not attacked before the 29th of June 1862. Then four gunboats tested the strength of the work and the efficiency of its garrison—the DeKalb Riflemen, Captain A. L. Hartridge. The first they found to be strong and the latter cool and very accurate in their aim. In this attack two men were wounded. On the 2d of November of the same year the fort was again made a target of by several vessels. Fortunately none of the garrison (the Emmett rifles, Captain George A. Nicoll) were hurt. This attack was followed by another on the 19th of November, during which three men of the garrison (the Emmett Rifles and the Republican Blues, Lieutenant Geo. W. Anderson commanding) were wounded. The 27th of January, 1863, was taken advantage of by the Federals to try the effect of the guns (one fifteen and one eleven-inch) of the ironclad Montauk. The monitor was accompanied by six gunboats, all of which kept up a furious fire, to which the garrison slowly replied. Though the sand of which the work was composed was knocked about considerably, none of the garrison were injured, nor was the earthwork at all damaged, thus demonstrating that an earthwork manned by cool and courageous men could not be reduced, no matter what weight of metal was hurled against it. The garrison had little respite, for on the first of February it had to defend the fort from another attack made by the Montauk and five gun and mortar boats. The enemy were again repulsed after a six hours contest, during which Major John B. Gallie* (commandant

* Major Gallie was a native of Scotland, and was fifty-six years of age when killed. He was a gallant soldier and a sincere christian. His loss was deeply deplored. Previous to the war he was in business in Savannah, a partner of the firm of Wilder & Gallie.

of the fort) was struck on the head and instantly killed, and seven others of the garrison were wounded. After the death of Major Gallie, which occurred early in the action, the command devolved upon Captain George W. Anderson, who bravely continued the fight with the result stated. Well deserved was the following complimentary order from General Beauregard: "The thanks of the country are due to this intrepid garrison, who have thus shown what brave men may withstand and accomplish, despite apparent odds. Fort McAllister will be inscribed on the flags of all the troops engaged in the defence of the battery."

On the 28th of February the Rattlesnake (formerly the Nashville), laden with a large quantity of cotton and rosin, attempted to pass down the Great Ogeechee, in order to run the blockade, but unfortunately ran aground about a mile below the fort. The guns of the Montauk were immediately brought to bear and soon set the vessel on fire, by which she was completely destroyed. The guns of the fort were fired at the Montauk, with the hope of driving her off, but the distance was too great and no damage was done. But what the guns failed to do was accomplished by a torpedo, over which the Montauk passed and exploded it during the attack upon the Rattlesnake. As she did not take any active part in the attack upon the fort a few days afterward, it was believed that she was injured, which belief was afterward confirmed by Northern accounts.

But the most formidable attack on the fort was made on the 3d of March, 1863, in comparison to which the others were almost insignificant. Early on that day four ironclads, five gunboats, and two mortar schooners appeared in front of the fort. From the account of the affair in the Savannah Republican of the 11th of March, 1863, we make the following extracts:

> About a quarter before nine o'clock the fort opened on the Passaic with a rifled gun, the eight and ten-inch columbiads following suit, to which the Montauk replied, firing her first gun at nine o'clock. She was followed by her associates in quick succession. The fire on both sides was continued for seven hours and a half, during which the enemy fired two hundred and fifty shot and shell at the fort, amounting to about seventy tons of the most formidable missiles ever invented for the destruction of human life. * * * About midday the carriage of the eight-inch columbiad was shivered to atoms and rendered the gun unserviceable for the remainder of the day. The main traverse wheel of the forty-two-pounder was shot away, but was replaced in twenty minutes. The new wheel was gotten up by Mr. Carroll Hanson, who risked his life to secure it. The wheel of a thirty-two-pounder, manned

by a detachment of sharpshooters, under the command of Lieutenant Herman, met with a similar accident, but was worked throughout the engagement. * * A shot from a forty-two-pounder struck the Passaic and disabled her, causing her to turn tail and run down the river, followed by the other rams. The fort fired the first and last shot. The enemy's mortar boats kept up a fire all night, and it was evidently their intention to renew the fight the next morning, but finding that the damage done to the fort the day before had been fully repaired and the garrison fully prepared to resist, declined. * * * Notwithstanding the heavy fire to which the fort was subjected, only three men were wounded, viz: Thomas W. Rape and W. S. Owens, of the Emmett Rifles, the first on the knee and the latter in the face; James Mims, of Company D, 1st Georgia Battalion Sharpshooters, had his leg crushed and ankle broken by the fall of a piece of timber while remounting a columbiad after the fight. * * * The night previous to the fight Lieutenant E. A. Ellarbe, of the Hardwick Mounted Rifles, Captain J. L. McAllister, with a detachment consisting of Sergeant Harmon and privates Proctor, Wyatt, Harper, and Cobb, crossed the river and dug a rifle-pit within long rifle range of the rams, and awaited the coming fight. During the hottest part of the engagement an officer, with glass in hand, made his appearance on the deck of the Passaic. A Maynard rifle slug soon went whizzing by his ears, which startled and caused him to right-about, when a second slug apparently took effect upon his person, as with both hands he caught hold of the turret for support, and immediately clambered or was dragged into a port-hole. It is believed that the officer was killed. The display on the Passaic the day following, and the funeral on Ossabaw the Friday following, gave strength to the opinion. As soon as the fatal rifle shot was fired the Passaic turned her guns upon the marsh and literally raked it with grapeshot. The riflemen, however, succeeded in changing their base in time to avoid the missiles of the enemy. Not one of them was hurt. Too much credit cannot be bestowed on this daring act of a few brave men. * * * Captain George W. Anderson, of the Republican Blues, commanded the fort on this trying occasion, and he and his force received, as they deserved, the highest commendations. Captain George A. Nicoll, of the Emmett Rifles; Captain J. L. McAllister, Lieutenant W. D. Dixon, and Sergeant T. S. Flood [the latter was sick at the hospital when the attack commenced, but left his bed to take part in the fight]; Corporal Robert Smith and his squad from the Republican Blues, which worked the rifle-gun; Lieutenant Quinn, of the Blues; Sergeant Frazier, Lieutenant Rockwell, and Sergeant Cavanagh; Captain Robert Martin and detachment of his company, who successfully worked a mortar-battery; Captain McCrady and Captain James McAlpin; were entitled to and received a large share of the honors of the day.

Brigadier-General Mercer, commanding the district of Georgia, in a general order, complimented the garrison for their heroic defence, stating that under the fire of the most formidable missiles ever concentrated upon a single battery "the brave gunners, with the cool, efficient spirit of disciplined soldiers, and with the intrepid hearts of freemen battling in a just cause, stood undaunted at their posts and proved to the world that the most formidable vessels and guns that modern ingenuity has been able to produce are powerless against an earthwork manned by patriots to whom honor and liberty are dearer than life."

General Beauregard in his general order stated that he "had again a pleasant duty to discharge—to commend to the notice of the country and the emulation of his officers and men the intrepid conduct of the garrison of Fort McAllister and the skill of the officers engaged on the 3d of March, 1863. * * * The colors of all troops engaged will be inscribed with 'Fort McAllister, 3d March, 1863.'"

After this engagement the fort was considerably strengthened—especially its rear defences—and its armament increased by the addition of some heavy and several light guns. The latter were so placed as to aid in repulsing any attempt of the enemy to surprise the fort from the land side.

On the 11th of December, 1864, General Sherman's army enveloped the western and southern lines of the defences of the city and completely isolated the fort, the garrison then consisting of the Emmett Rifles, Captain George A. Nicoll, twenty-five men for duty; Clinch Light Battery, Captain W. B. Clinch, fifty men for duty; Companies D and E 1st regiment Georgia Reserves, the first company commanded by Captain Henry, twenty-eight men for duty, and the second by Captain Morrison, twenty-seven men for duty. On the 13th of December General Hazen was sent with nine regiments to take the fort.

Major George W. Anderson was in command of the fort at the time of its capture, and furnished a report of the affair to Colonel C. C. Jones for publication in his "Historical Sketch of the Chatham Artillery," from which we extract it:

Hearing incidentally that the Confederate forces on the Cannouchee had evacuated that position and retired across the Great Ogeechee, and learning that a large column of the enemy was approaching in the direction of Fort McAllister, I immediately detached a scouting party, under command of Lieutenant T. O'Neal, of Clinch's Light Battery, to watch them and acquaint me with their movements. This was absolutely necessary, as the cavalry previously stationed in Bryan county had been withdrawn and I was thus thrown upon my own resources for all information relating to the strength and designs of the enemy.

On the morning of the 12th of December, 1864, I accompanied Lieutenant O'Neal on a scout, and found the enemy advancing in force from King's bridge. We were hotly pursued by their cavalry, and had barely time to burn the barns of Messrs. Thomas C. Arnold and William Patterson, which were filled with rice. The steamtug Columbus—lying about three miles above the fort—was also burned. Early the next morning one of my pickets—stationed at the head of the causeway west of the fort—was captured by the enemy, to whom he imparted the fact that the causeway was studded with torpedoes in time to prevent their explosion. He also acquainted them with the strength of the garrison, and the armament of the fort, and the best approaches to it.

About eight o'clock A. M. desultory firing commenced between the skirmishers of the enemy and my sharpshooters. At ten o'clock the fight became general, the opposing forces extending from the river entirely around to the marsh on the east. The day before, the enemy had established a battery of Parrot guns on the opposite side of the river—distant from the fort a mile and a half—which fired upon us at regular intervals during that day and the ensuing night. Receiving from headquarters neither orders nor responses to my telegraphic dispatches, I determined, under the circumstances, and notwithstanding the great disparity of numbers, between the garrison and the attacking forces, to defend the fort to the last extremity. The guns being *en barbette*, the detachments serving them were greatly exposed to the fire of the enemy's sharpshooters. To such an extent was this the case, that in one instance, out of a detachment of eight men, three were killed and three more wounded. The Federal skirmish line was very heavy, and the fire so close and rapid that it was at times impossible to work our guns. My sharpshooters did all in their power, but were entirely too few to suppress this galling fire upon the artillerists. In view of the large force of the enemy—consisting of nine regiments, whose aggregate strength was estimated between three thousand five hundred and four thousand muskets, and possessing the ability to increase it at any time should it become necessary—and recollecting the feebleness of the garrison of the fort, numbering one hundred and fifty effective men, it was evident, cut off from all support, and with no possible hope of reinforcements from any quarter, that holding the fort was simply a question of time. There was but one alternative—death or captivity. Captain Thomas S. White, the engineer in charge, had previously felled the trees in the vicinity of the fort, and demolished the mortar magazine which commanded the fort to a very considerable extent. For lack of the necessary force and time, however, the felled timber and the ruins of the adjacent houses, which had been pulled down, had not been entirely removed. Protected by this cover, the enemy's sharpshooters were enabled to approach quite near, to the great annoyance and injury of the cannoneers. One line of abattis had been constructed by the engineer, and three lines would have been completed around the fort, but for the want of time and material.

Late in the afternoon the full force of the enemy made a rapid and vigorous charge upon the works, and, succeeding in forcing their way through the abattis, rushed over the parapet of the fort, carrying it by storm, and, by virtue of superior numbers, overpowered the garrison, fighting gallantly to the last. In many instances the Confederates were disarmed by main force. *The fort was never surrendered. It was captured by overwhelming numbers.* So soon as the enemy opened fire upon the fort from the opposite side of the river, it was evident that two of the magazines were seriously endangered, and it became necessary to protect them from that fire by the erection of suitable traverses. The labor expended in their construction, in the mounting of guns on the rear of the work, and in removing the debris above referred to, occupied the garrison constantly, night and day, for nearly forty-eight hours immediately preceding the attack. Consequently, at the time of the assault, the men were greatly fatigued and in bad plight, physically considered, for the contest. I think it not improper to state here that a short time before the approach of the enemy a member of the torpedo department had, in obedience to orders, placed in front of the fort, and along the direct approaches, a considerable number of sub-terra shells, whose explosions killed quite a number of the enemy while passing over them.

After the capture of the fort, General Sherman in person ordered my engineer with a detail of sixteen men from the garrison—then prisoners of war—to remove all the torpedoes which had not exploded. This hazardous duty was performed without injury to any one; but it appearing to me to be an unwarrantable and improper treatment of prisoners of war, I have thought it right to refer to it in this report.

I am pleased to state that in my endeavors to hold the fort, I was nobly seconded by the great majority of officers and men under my command. Many of them had never been under fire before, and quite a number were very young, in fact mere boys. Where so many acted gallantly, it would be invidious to discriminate; but I cannot avoid mentioning those who came more particularly under my notice. I would therefore most respectfully call the attention of the General commanding to the gallant conduct of Captain Clinch, who, when summoned to surrender by a Federal Captain, responded by dealing him a severe blow on the head with his sabre. (Captain Clinch had previously received two gun-shot wounds in the arm.) Immediately a hand to hand fight ensued. Federal privates came to the assistance of their officer, but the fearless Clinch continued the unequal contest until he fell bleeding from eleven wounds (three sabre wounds, six bayonet wounds, and two gun-shot wounds), from which, after severe and protracted suffering, he has barely recovered. His conduct was so conspicuous, and his cool bravery so much admired, as to elicit the praise of the enemy and even of General Sherman himself.

1st Lieutenant William Schirm fought his guns until the enemy had entered the fort, and notwithstanding a wound in the head, gallantly remained at his post, discharging his duties with a coolness and efficiency worthy of all commendation.

Lieutenant O'Neal, whom I placed in command of the scouting party before mentioned, while in the discharge of that duty, and in his subsequent conduct during the attack, merited the honor due to a faithful and gallant officer.

Among those who nobly fell was the gallant Hazzard, whose zeal and activity were worthy of all praise. He died as a true soldier to his post, facing overwhelming odds. The garrison lost seventeen killed and thirty-one wounded.

A Federal officer in writing an account of the siege of Savannah and storming of Fort McAllister said:

Those were dark days when the marching was over and the army had settled down in the flooded forests and before the frowning fortifications of Savannah.

Notwithstanding the orders to forage upon the enemy on the way, the thirty days' rations were in parts of the army exhausted when it came to the halt, where there was no food except such as the rice-fields afforded. Then for the first time the confident cheerfulness of the chief gave place to deep thought and anxious preoccupation. It required several days for the army to establish its position. By turning aside the waters of the canal which united the swift current of the Savannah with its sluggish sister, the Ogeechee, the low swamp-lands were covered neck-deep by the treacherous element; and where the raised causeways spanned these forest bogs the enemy had girded them about with fort and bastion. Every attempt in these places to push forward our lines met with the fire of heavy artillery and the blazing sheets of infantry flame. It was not the city of Savannah our commander coveted in those days of 1864 so much as bread. Sherman might not with the hapless Queen of France answer the cry for food with "Give them bonbons!" and so he sought for the sea.

* * * * * * * * * * *

Weeks before, while the army was yet among the hills of Georgia, some soldier, while rumaging among a package of letters which he had found in a house by the road-side, came upon a scrap of thin brown paper, marked with curved lines, which to the ordinary eye would have been meaningless; but to any intelligent American soldier, who had used pick and shovel, it had interest and significance. The writing on this paper ran something in this way:

DEAR MOTHER: Here I am in a big fort way off on the Ogeechee river. It is called Fort McAllister, which is the name of a plantation hereabouts. It is a big fort with thirty or forty big guns, which we fire at the Yankee vessels whenever they come up the river. They have tried it on with ironclads and all that, but we always beat them off, and are perfectly safe behind our tall bomb-proofs. You can't imagine how crooked this river is—a snake wriggling is a straight line compared to it. I send you a little drawing which I have made of the bend in the river and the position of the fort. A strong place it is, and the Yanks never can take it so long as they knock at the front door. * * * We don't have much to eat, and it's right lonely here. * * * * * *

The soldier gave this bit of paper to his captain, and it so came on through General Howard to General Sherman; and as he carefully examined it I remember hearing some one say: "Fort McAllister! I never heard of such a place before. It must be one of the rebel line of sea defences." * * * *

Hazen's troops, the general carrying in his pocket the slip of brown paper which many months ago the rebel soldier had sent to his mother way up in Georgia, halted not at tangled abattis, they did not heed the torpedoes exploding under their feet, but plunged into the deep ditch, tore away the tough palisades, mounted to the parapet, and there, then, and within the fort, fought hand to hand with its gallant defenders; and when the smoke, painfully lifting itself into the heavy air of evening, revealed the flag of our Union planted there, we, envious and impatient lookers-on, knew that victory was inscribed all over its beautiful folds.

To Hazen the capture of Fort McAllister was glory, undying fame. To the Commander-in-chief it meant bread, food, the conquest of Savannah. How swift moved events when the brazen door to the sea was unlocked! And first and most important was the feast of hard tack; and a more welcome feast was never offered to a hungry host since the days the children of Israel found manna in the wilderness. The destructive torpedoes in the river were released from their moorings, and scores of busy, puffing steam-tugs paddled up the stream, loaded with precious freight of bread. There was enough, more than enough, for all. Bread for man and food for beast. Profane fellows, who had well-nigh forgotten how to pray, now offered up grateful thanks. The soldier in his rifle-pit heeded not the mud and water, and patted his ration of hard bread with loving tenderness. As the wagons creaked into camp, groaning with their cargo of white boxes filled with hard tack, the eager groups of hungry men surrounded them with cheers of welcome. The army of refugees, crouching in their miserable camps among the bushes, were not forgotten.

After the fall of Fort McAllister both armies lay comparatively idle, awaiting what was shortly expected to be bloody work. The enemy made numerous feints of storming our works, but hostile operations were mainly confined to petty skirmishes.* The enemy, as was admitted after the surrender by a Colonel of their army, attempted to throw shell into the city, no warning of such intention being given. The Colonel stated that his gunners, in a battery on the west of the city, had their guns double-charged, hoping that the extra load would hurl the shells into the city. One shell fell near the Central Railroad bridge, and another into the river one hundred yards above the upper rice-mill. On the 19th of December the enemy placed an army corps on the South Carolina shore with a view of cutting off the Confederate army should they attempt to retreat. All hope of successfully coping with the powerful force of the enemy was rightly abandoned by General Hardee, and he concluded to evacuate the city and thus save his command to the Confederacy. A pontoon bridge was laid across the river from Anderson's wharf, a few paces west of Barnard street, to Hutchinson's island, and another one from thence to the South Carolina shore. Early on the 20th a small force was sent over and dislodged a body of the enemy's troops posted across a road by which the proposed retreat was to be made. At night the Confederates were quietly withdrawn from the intrenchments, marched through the city, across the pontoon bridges into South Carolina, and safely escaped up the country. All the artillery and stores that could be removed were carried off. A large number of families left during the night in private conveyances, following the retreating troops.

The members of the council were notified by the commander of his intention to evacuate the city, and a special meeting was called.

---

* It being reported that General Sherman made two demands for the surrender of Savannah, we wrote repeatedly to the Confederate officers who could have correctly informed us in this regard, but received no reply.—EDS.

While the troops were leaving the city Dr. R. D. Arnold, Mayor, and Aldermen Henry Brigham, J. F. O'Byrne, C. C. Casey, Henry Freeman, Robert Lachlison, Joseph Lippman, J. L. Villalonga, and George W. Wylly met in the Exchange and resolved that the Council should repair to the outer defences before daylight, to surrender the city and secure such terms as would ensure protection to the persons and property of the citizens from the soldiers whose previous conduct filled the minds of all with a lively apprehension that slaughter and rapine would mark their entrance into the city. The council dispersed to assemble at the Exchange at a later hour, where hacks would await to convey the members to the outer works. As they came out of the Exchange a fire was observed in the western part of the city, and, by request, Messrs. Casey, O'Byrne, and Lachlison went to it with a view of taking measures for its suppression. The fire was caused by the burning of a nearly-completed ironclad and a lot of timber near the mouth of the Ogeechee canal which had been fired by the retreating troops. The wind was blowing to the west, and after observing that no danger to the city need be apprehended from the flames these gentlemen returned to the Exchange, where the other members of the Council had assembled and were in a hack prepared to start. They stated that other hacks had been provided, but General Wheeler's cavalry had pressed the horses into service. Mr. O'Byrne procured his horse and buggy and conveyed Mr. Casey to the junction of the Lewisburg road with the Augusta road—about half of a mile beyond the Central Railroad depot—and leaving him there returned for Mr. Lachlison, who had walked in that direction. The party in the hack, meanwhile, had come up to Mr. Casey, and taking him up drove up the Lewisburg road. Mr. O'Byrne met Mr. Lachlison, and with him returned to where Mr. Casey had been left, but not finding any of the party there, concluded they had gone up the Augusta road, and proceeded up it, hoping to overtake them. They advanced but a short distance when they heard the report of a gun and a minnie ball whistled between them. They halted, and were then ordered by the pickets to turn around (they had unawares passed the enemy's picket and had not heard the command to halt) and come to them. They did as commanded, and after informing the officer of the picket who they were, were conducted to Colonel Barnum, to whom they stated the object of their mission. He then conducted them to General John W. Geary. They told him that the city had been evacuated, and that they, having started with the Mayor and Council to surrender it, but became separated from them, would assume the authority of consummating a surrender. General Geary at first did not believe them, and questioned them very closely. After becoming satisfied that they were what they assumed to be, he consented to receive the surrender. The Aldermen then asked that the lives and property of the citizens should be respected and the ladies protected from insult. General Geary promptly replied that the requests should be complied with, and that any soldier detected violating the orders which would be given to restrain them should be punished with death. Messrs. Lachlison and O'Byrne then asked that a detachment should be sent to look after the Mayor and other Aldermen, which was granted. General Geary then put his troops in motion and, with Messrs. O'Byrne and Lachlison acting as guides, advanced toward the city. At the Central Railroad bridge they were met by the Mayor and Aldermen, who had been overtaken by the detachment sent for them and returned with it. They, on being introduced to the General and being told of what had been done by Messrs. O'Byrne and Lachlison, confirmed their action. The line of march was then taken up to West Broad street, down that to the Bay, and thence to the Exchange, in front of which the troops were drawn up. The officers and the members of the Council proceeded to the porch, from which General Geary addressed the troops, complimenting them upon their past deeds and upon the additional honor they had conferred upon themselves by capturing "this beautiful city of the South." During this speech Colonel Barnum observed a sergeant step out of the ranks to the store at the corner of Bull and Bay streets—now occupied by Messrs. Gazan & Bro.—enter and come out wearing a fireman's hat. On coming down from the porch he called the sergeant to him, and drawing his sword ordered him to hold out the hat, which he did, and the Colonel with one stroke of his sword cut it in half. He then stripped the chevrons from the sergeant's arms and reduced him to the ranks.

After the speech the troops were dispersed in squads throughout the city, and notwithstanding the strict orders they had received committed many depredations; among them the wanton destruction of valuable books and papers in the Exchange and Courthouse belonging to the city and county. General Geary established his headquarters in the Central Railroad bank and his subordinate officers in the various unoccupied stores along the Bay. On the

24th of December he issued an order regarding the posts and duties of the provost guards, and instructing the civil authorities to resume their official duties.

General W. T. Sherman arrived in the city on the 25th, and after telegraphing President Lincoln that he would present him Savannah as a "Christmas gift," promulgated the following order from his headquarters at the Green mansion, opposite Oglethorpe Barracks. The order speaks for itself:

HEADQUARTERS MILITARY DIVISION OF THE MISSISSIPPI,
In the Field, Savannah, Georgia, December 26th, 1864.

SPECIAL FIELD ORDERS,
No. 143.

The City of Savannah and surrounding country will be held as a Military Post and adapted to future military uses, but as it contains a population of some 20,000 people who must be provided for, and as other citizens may come, it is proper to lay down certain general principles, that all within its military jurisdiction may understand their relative duties and obligations.

I. During War, the Military is superior to Civil authority, and where interests clash, the Civil must give way, yet where there is no conflict, every encouragement should be given to well-disposed and peaceful inhabitants to resume their usual pursuits. Families should be disturbed as little as possible in their residences, and tradesmen allowed the free use of their shops, tools, &c. Churches, schools, all places of amusement and recreation should be encouraged, and streets and roads made perfectly safe to persons in their usual pursuits. Passes should not be exacted within the line of outer pickets, but if any person shall abuse these privileges by communicating with the enemy, or doing any act of hostility to the Government of the United States, he or she will be punished with the utmost rigor of the law.

Commerce with the outer world will be resumed to an extent commensurate with the wants of the citizens, governed by the restrictions and rules of the Treasury Department.

II. The Chief Quartermaster and Commissary of the Army may give suitable employment to the people, white or black, or transport them to such points as they choose, where employment may be had, and may extend temporary relief in the way of provisions and vacant houses to the worthy and needy until such time as they can help themselves. They will select first, the buildings for the necessary uses of the army; next a sufficient number of stores to be turned over to the Treasury Agent for trade stores. All vacant store-houses or dwellings, and all buildings belonging to absent rebels, will be construed and used as belonging to the United States until such times as their titles can be settled by the Courts of the United States.

III. The Mayor and City Council of Savannah will continue to exercise their functions as such, and will, in concert with the Commanding Officer of the Post and the Chief Quartermaster, see that the Fire Companies are kept in organization, the streets cleaned and lighted, and keep up a good understanding between the citizens and soldiers. They will ascertain and report to the Chief C. S., as soon as possible, the names and number of worthy families that need assistance and support.

The Mayor will forthwith give public notice that the time has come when all must choose their course, viz: to remain within our lines and conduct themselves as good citizens or depart in peace. He will ascertain the names of all who choose to leave Savannah, and report their names and residences to the Chief Quartermaster, that measures may be taken to transport them beyond the lines.

IV. Not more than two Newspapers will be published in Savannah, and their Editors and Proprietors will be held to the strictest accountability, and will be punished severely in person and property for any libellous publication, mischievous matter, premature news, exaggerated statements, or any comments whatever upon the acts of the constituted authorities; they will be held accountable even for such articles though copied from other papers.

By Order of Major-General W. T. SHERMAN.

L. M. DRAYTON, Aide-de-Camp.

A meeting of the citizens was held in the Masonic hall on the 28th of December, to "take into consideration matters appertaining to the present and future welfare of the city." Dr. R. D. Arnold presided. The following preamble and resolutions were adopted:

WHEREAS, By the fortunes of war and the surrender of the city by the civil authorities, the city of Savannah passes once more under the authority of the United States; and whereas, we believe that the interests of the city will be best subserved and promoted by a full and free expression of our views in relation to our present condition; we, therefore, the People of Savannah in full meeting assembled do hereby resolve:

That we accept the position, and in the language of the President of the United States, seek to have "peace by laying down our arms and submitting to the National authority under the Constitution, leaving all questions which remain to be adjusted by the peaceful means of legislation, conference and votes."

Resolved, That laying aside all differences, and burying by-gones in the grave of the past, we will use our best endeavors once more to bring back the prosperity and commerce we once enjoyed.

Resolved, That we do not put ourselves in the position of a conquered city, asking terms of a conqueror, but we claim the immunities and privileges contained in the Proclamation and Message of the President of the United States and in all the legislation of Congress in reference to a people situated as we are, and while we owe on our part a strict obedience to the laws of the United States, we ask the protection over our persons, lives and property recognized by these laws.

On the night of the 31st of December the blockade-runner Rebecca Hertz, Captain King, "ran the blockade" (as the crew thought, not knowing of the change which had recently taken place in the government of the city) and dropped anchor opposite the gas-house. Daylight revealed the fact that the stars and stripes were fluttering at the points from which a short time before floated the stars and bars. This somewhat amazed the blockade-runners, but the situation was taken in at a glance, and Captain King turned his vessel over to the Quartermaster's Department.

Shortly after this occurrence Sherman started a corps across our pontoon bridges into South Carolina. While a large number of the soldiers were delayed on Hutchinson's island the river rose very rapidly. The troops rushed back for the city, but a number of the men and horses were drowned in attempting to reach the bridge.

Among the first acts of the Federal troops after their arrival in Savannah was the throwing up of intrenchments to resist any attempt of the Confederates to recapture the city. They also threw up intrenchments on the Thunderbolt road, and mounted guns to bear upon the city. This was intended as a rallying point if they were driven from the other intrenchments. With a heartlessness for which there is no palliation, not even that of "military necessity," they ran this line of works through the Catholic Cemetery, destroying, mutilating, or covering up the monuments and tablets which the hand of affection had placed over the graves of the loved and lost, and in numerous instances dug up the bones and left them scattered about. It was asserted by the officers, when remonstrated with for their inhumanity in desecrating the graves, that the work was necessary, and would not have been done had it not been a "military necessity." There was no more necessity for it than there was for the breaking open of the vaults in the Old Burying-ground and at Bonaventure, in search of valuables which the soldiers supposed were hidden in them.

The shock occasioned by the fall of Savannah was being rapidly recovered from, under what appeared to be the mild and just administration of affairs by the military, and all hoped for a speedy restoration of quiet and prosperity, even though under military rule. But alas! these expectations were doomed to meet with disappointment. The mildness and justness which had characterized the conquerors upon their first arrival were reversed, and a series of unjust acts and petty persecutions commenced.

When the city was evacuated there were thirty thousand five hundred bales of upland and a little over eight thousand bales of sea island cotton stored in the warehouses, only one thousand bales of which belonged to the Confederate States government. Under the pretence that the cotton belonged to the Confederate government, the United States Quartermasters seized all of it (and a large quantity of other property also) and shipped it to New York, where uplands commanded one dollar and twenty-five cents and sea island three dollars per pound, making the total value of the cotton seized about twenty-eight millions of dollars. It was stored in New York, where, in the meaning of General Sherman's order, it remained, to "be construed and used as belonging to the United States until such times as their titles can be settled by the Courts of the United States;" (i. e., what time has shown, after the claimants have spent in court and lawyers' fees the value of the cotton claimed). Citizens were not allowed to pass through the streets in their daily pursuits without a pass which they had to show at the bidding of every insolent and drunken officer or soldier who, whether on or off duty, felt disposed to exercise the power granted him by the bayonet. No one, ladies not excepted, could receive a letter from the postoffice unless he or she had taken the oath. Added to these petty tyrannies was the unbridled conduct of the negroes and soldiers, which kept the timid in a perpetual state of alarm.

While thus harassed and depressed the people were called upon to bear another calamity—the fire on the night of the 27th of January, 1865—which destroyed over a hundred buildings, and threatened the destruction of the entire city. To the usual horrors of an extensive fire was added the dangers of a terrific bombardment. The fire—supposed to have been the work of the soldiers of the 20th United States Army corps,* and the beginning of an organized attempt to set fire to the city, as during the night fire was discovered in St. Andrews' hall, in the Exchange, and at other places throughout the city—commenced in a stable in the rear of the old "Granite hall" (located at the corner of West Broad and Zubly streets), which had been used by the Confederate authorities as an arsenal for fixed ammunition, and in which there were stored thousands of rounds. The fire spread rapidly. Citizens and soldiers crowded to the scene, and under orders of an United States officer, commenced to remove the ammunition and assist in

* The soldiers of this corps believed that they would be detailed to remain in Savannah when Sherman's army advanced, which occurred on this night. Another corps was detailed, and much ill feeling sprung up between the corps, and it was the belief of the soldiers of the corps detailed to remain that the other corps attempted to destroy the city to prevent the necessity of their remaining.

working the engines. Before much of the ammunition had been removed the fire was communicated to the powder, and explosion after explosion followed in rapid succession, the fragments of shell flying in all directions, killing a negro and wounding two or three citizens. Pieces of shell were picked up near the Pulaski and also the Greene monument, and in the yards of citizens living in remote parts of the city. The first explosion scattered the crowd and aroused those asleep, many of whom, before realizing the state of affairs, thought the Confederate troops had made a night attack. During this novel bombardment, which put a stop to the working of the engines in the vicinity and allowed the fire full sway, a piece of shell struck the reservoir. A jet of water immediately sprung out, which for novelty and beauty surpassed any fountain, looking in the fiery glare like a sheet of molten silver. Before the flames were arrested over one hundred houses, situated on West Broad between Pine and St. Gaul streets, and a few on Broughton and Congress streets, were destroyed.

The crowning act of oppression was yet to come—that of removing the families of the officers of the Confederate army and navy out of the city. When all the other deeds of rapine, murder, and oppression which have been laid at the door of General Sherman have been buried in the dust of oblivion, this will remain a reproach and a disgrace to him who, not many years before, when a lieutenant at Oglethorpe barracks, was hospitably entertained by the relatives of the ladies who, with their children, he now had torn away from their friends and sent into the Confederate lines, knowing full well that they must inevitably suffer from want and exposure before meeting again with their lawful protectors. What occasioned this action is not known. Perhaps General Sherman* had read of the British sending ladies from Savannah during the Revolutionary war, and did not desire to be outdone by them in cruelty and oppression. Whatever may have been the occasion, he or his subordinates never published an order defining his reasons or notifying the ladies publicly that they must leave, but sent word privately by staff officers that it was the intention of the commander to remove them, and that they must register their names by a certain

* It is stated that Edward M. Stanton, United States Secretary of War, who came to Savannah shortly after its evacuation, ordered that the wives and children of the Confederate officers should be sent out of the city, against which Sherman at first demurred, but afterward consented, and gave the necessary commands to have the order carried out.

time. It appears that all did not register, or at least not as many as Brevet Major-General C. Grover, then in command of Savannah, thought should have done so, and he published the following order, the italics appearing in it:

[CIRCULAR.]

OFFICE PROVOST MARSHAL, DISTRICT SAVANNAH,
March 28th, 1865.

The wives and families of Confederate officers who have not registered their names at this office *will do so at once.*

By order of Brevet Major-General C. GROVER, commanding.

ROBERT P. YORK,
Provost Marshal District Savannah, Ga.

On the 31st of March the ladies and children were placed on board of the steamer Hudson, to be carried under flag of truce to Augusta. Arriving at Sister's ferry, about sixty-four miles from Savannah, the boat stopped and the captain refused to proceed further up the river. General Edward C. Anderson, commanding at that point, had the ladies and children transferred to the shore and transported them to Augusta in wagons, the only means of conveyance at hand.

Shortly after this disgraceful affair the armies of Generals Lee and Johnston surrendered; the loved and honored and saved returned to cheer their old places with their presence; the restrictions upon commerce and business were gradually removed, a partial civil government restored, and under the blessings of a divine providence peace, prosperity, and plenty returned. Four years have now elapsed since the capture of the city, and Savannah is larger and more prosperous than before the war.

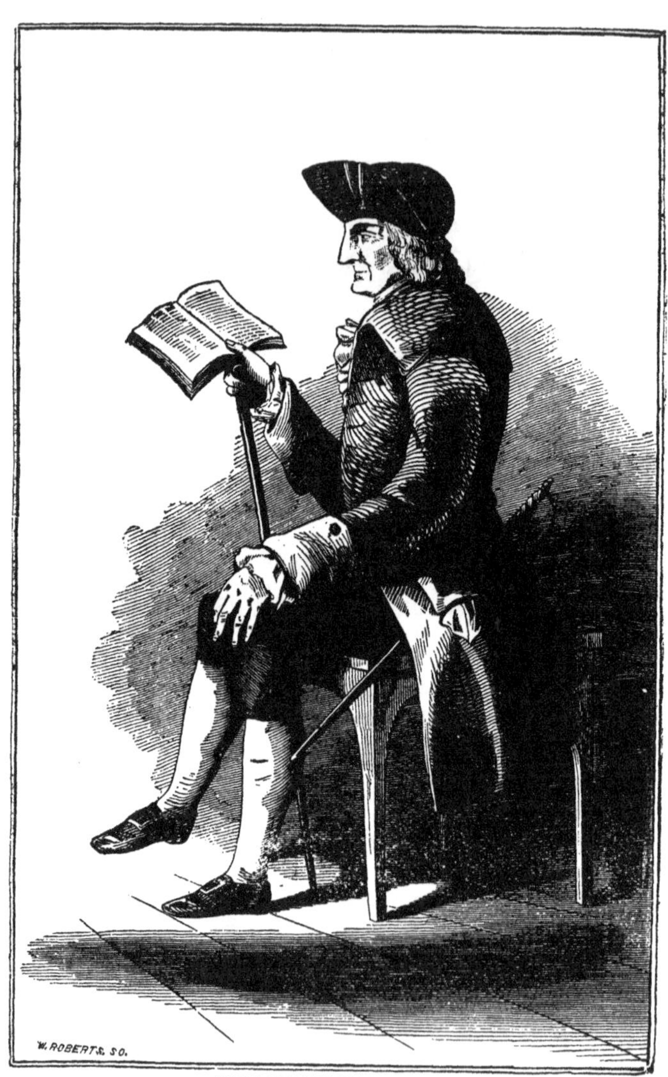

JAMES EDWARD OGLETHORPE.

JAMES EDWARD OGLETHORPE,

THE FOUNDER OF SAVANNAH, GA.,

Was born in London on the 21st of December, 1688. At the age of sixteen he was admitted a student of the Corpus Christi college, but did not finish his studies—the military profession having more charms for him than literary pursuits. His first commission was that of ensign. After the death of Queen Anne he entered into the service of Prince Eugene. He entered Parliament at the age of twenty-four, and continued a member thirty-two years. He established the colony at Savannah in 1733. In 1743 he left for England to answer some charges preferred against him by Lieutenant-Colonel Cook for alleged mismanagement during the war with the Spaniards. A court-martial declared the charges groundless and malicious, and Cook was dismissed from service. In 1744 Oglethorpe was appointed one of the field officers under Field Marshal the Earl of Stair, to oppose the expected invasion of the French. Well might a cotemporaneous writer of him say that he "doubts whether the histories of Greece or Rome can produce a greater instance of public spirit than this. To see a gentleman of his rank and fortune visiting a distant and uncultivated land, with no other society but the unfortunate whom he goes to assist, exposing himself freely to the same hardships to which they are subjected, in the prime of life, instead of pursuing his pleasures or ambition, on an improved and well-concerted plan from which his country must reap the profits; at his own expense, and without a view or even a possibility of receiving any private advantage from it; this, too, after having done and expended for what many generous men would think sufficient to have done—to see this, I say, must give every one who has approved and contributed to the undertaking the highest satisfaction; must convince the world of the disinterested zeal with which the settlement is to be made and entitle him to the highest honor he can gain—the perpetual love and applause of mankind." He died in England on the 1st of July, 1785.

CHAPTER VIII.

Biographical Sketch of General Francis S. Bartow— Brief Historical Records of the Volunteer Companies of Savannah: Chatham Artillery — Georgia Hussars (companies A and B) — Savannah Volunteer Guards (companies A, B, and C) — Republican Blues — Phœnix Riflemen (companies A, B, and C) — Irish Jasper Greens (companies A and B) — German Volunteers — Oglethorpe Light Infantry (companies A and B) — Irish Volunteers (companies A and B) — Washington Volunteers — Blue Cap Cavalry — City Light Guard — Savannah Cadets — Montgomery Guards — Mitchell Volunteer Guards — DeKalb Riflemen — Emmett Rifles — Oglethorpe Siege Artillery — Tatnall Guards — Coast Rifles.

It is meet that the record of the officers and soldiers of Savannah, whose deeds on the many battle-fields of the South illustrated the prowess of Southern chivalry, should commence with a biographical sketch of the life of General Francis S. Bartow, whose heroic and lamented death upon the plains of Manassas called for and received the admiration and encomiums of both friends and foes.

Francis S. Bartow, son of Theodosius Bartow, was born in Savannah on the 6th of September, 1816. He graduated at Franklin college, at Athens, Ga., in 1835, with the highest honors of his class. He then became a student in the law office of Messrs. Berrien & Law, of Savannah, and afterward attended the Law school at New Haven, Conn. Here he completed his studies, and shortly afterward was admitted to the bar and became a member of the well-known law firm of Law, Bartow & Lovell, of Savannah. His first forensic effort was in a great bank case, in which he greatly distinguished himself by the logical force and clearness of his argument and the power of his eloquence.

His political career commenced with the celebrated Harrison campaign in 1840, in which he took an active and influential part in the support of General Harrison, the Whig candidate for President. He was afterward elected to the State Senate, and served several times in the House of Representatives. During the later political contests he was not connected with political life. In 1860, when the impending storm produced the commotion in the political atmosphere, telling of the approaching revolution, his clear-seeing intellect convinced him that it must be resisted or his State would be crushed, and with that boldness and earnestness characteristic of him he placed himself in the very vanguard, and there remained until he consecrated his devotion to the new-born Confederacy by a generous outpouring of his life-blood.

He was the unanimous choice of the people of Chatham county to represent them in the State convention, which carried Georgia out of the Union, and among that body of able and patriotic men none more than he contributed to place his native State in the noble attitude of resistance to Federal thraldom. He was selected by the convention to represent the State in the Confederate Congress, which met in Montgomery, Alabama, and chosen chairman of the Military committee. While there, when differences of opinion arose regarding the course of action necessary to keep pace with the rapid march of mighty events, he boldly stood forward for firm and immediate action—bold and undaunted when the time came for him to act; modest and retiring under all other circumstances.

During the session of Congress he announced his intention to go to Virginia with his company, the Oglethorpe Light Infantry, of which he had been elected captain in 1857. He offered the company's services for the war to the President through Governor Brown, who refused to give his permission for them to leave, and Bartow then offered its services directly to the President, who accepted them. He returned to Savannah, and on the 21st of May, 1861, with his company, departed for the seat of war. His departure was made the occasion of a most scurrilous attack from Governor Brown (which was published in the papers throughout the State), charging him with disobedience of orders, with unlawfully carrying off the muskets belonging to the State, and of unpatriotic motives. Bartow's reply (published in the Savannah Morning News), was made in the following frank, manly, and dignified manner, triumphantly vindicating his motives and conduct:

CAMP DEFIANCE, HARPER'S FERRY,
June 14th, 1861.

To Governor JOSEPH E. BROWN:

Sir—I received your letter of the 21st of May ult., while at Richmond. Since the date of its reception I have been so constantly engaged in the duties of the service I have undertaken that I have found no time which could be devoted to an acknowledgment of your communication. I now write amidst the hurry and confusion of the camp, being about to march from this point, we trust, to meet the enemy.

I have little time and less inclination to reply in detail to the insolent missive you thought proper to publish in my absence. Respect, however, for the good opinion of the people of Georgia induces me in a few words to set right my conduct, which you have taken so much pains to asperse, and to correct the mis-statements and false imputations with which your letter abounds.

You say that I have "commenced my military career by setting at defiance the orders of the officer upon whom the Constitution of my State has conferred the right to command me." I am not aware that you have any such right, unless I were actually enlisted in the service of the State of Georgia, in a contingency which, under the Constitution, would give the State the right to raise and maintain troops.

I commenced my military career, as you are pleased to term it, under the flag of the Confederate States, and I recognize not *you, but the President of the Confederate States as the officer* upon whom the Constitution (to which Georgia is a party) "has conferred the right to command me." It is true that I tendered, under instructions from my company, their services to the Confederate States through you, in the first instance; this, however, was simply because the President had adopted that mode of obtaining troops as a matter of public convenience and *not because there ever was* any Constitution or law which *required* him to appeal to the State Executives; still less is there any ground for your assertion that the rights of the States are violated by the President receiving troops directly, without the intervention of the Governors.

You labor, and have constantly labored, under the impression that you are the State of Georgia. I beg leave to protest against this conclusion, in which I assure you I can never concur. By the Constitution of the Confederate States, to which Georgia has agreed, the Confederate Government is *alone* chargeable with questions of peace and war, and has the exclusive right, except in case of invasion, to raise and maintain armies. The Congress, and not the Governors of the States, are empowered to raise these armies: and as the constitution is broad and unqualified in this grant of power, the Congress is unrestricted in the mode in which it shall be exercised. The President of the Confederate States is the Commander-in-chief of these armies, thus raised for a common cause, and the Governors of States have not, so far as I am aware, any jurisdiction or power over this subject, *except* so far as patriotism may induce them to co-operate with the General Government in times of great emergency and danger. Your conclusion, therefore, that "the act of Congress under which I go is a palpable encroachment upon the rights of States" does not in the least disturb me. Neither upon reason nor authority do I consider the opinion of much value. I think most people will prefer the judgment of the Confederate Congress and the President of the Confederate States, who gave the act their deliberate sanction.

You have fallen into another error upon this subject. You say "that I proceeded to the Confederate Congress, of which I am a member, and, that a bill was passed, you suppose chiefly by my influence, which authorized the President to receive military forces over the head and independent of State authority." You further say that "under this act I was accepted into service without your consent and permitted to leave Savannah and go to Virginia." I assure you, in passing, that I shall never think it necessary to obtain *your* consent to enter the service of my country. God forbid that I should ever fall so low.

But to your charge. I know not to what act you refer as the one under which I was accepted into service; but I will inform you that the act under which I serve is entitled "An act to raise additional forces to *serve during the war.*" This act, to the best of my remembrance, contains no allusion to State authority, nor does it allude in any part to the Governors of States. It is simply an act authorizing the President to accept the services of volunteers for the war, and to appoint their field officers, and in these two respects alone, it differs from other acts under which volunteers have been accepted. This bill was introduced into Congress by the Hon. Mr. Wigfall, of Texas, without any consultation with me, referred to the Military committee, of which I was chairman, perfected by it and passed by the Congress. It met the approval of the most distinguished leaders of the States Rights school in the Congress, and was regarded by Congress as the best means to raise an efficient army, so absolutely required by the wicked invasion set on foot by the North. Mr. Wright, of Georgia, introduced a bill which does authorize the President, without calling upon the Governors of the States, to accept the services of volunteers at the times he may prescribe; but with this bill I had no connection, nor am I in service under its terms, nor had I any agency in procuring its introduction or enactment.

You go on to say "that I must be presumed to be the leading spirit in procuring the passage of this bill, and that I was the first to avail myself of its benefits by accepting a high command under it." You remark "that it is said I am to have a colonel's commission." Now, sir, the facts are, that under the former bill, by which twelve months' volunteers were raised for the war, the President had as much power to accept them directly as he had under this act, for the war; and it is a mere matter of discretion with him under both acts whether he will or will not use the intervention of State Executives; and yet, while stepping out of the way to stab me in the back, you seem criminally ignorant of what you ought to know.

You have also insinuated in this charge and elsewhere in your letter, that I have been misled by motives of personal ambition. The attribution of low motives of conduct to others is most frequently the result of long familiarity with such principles of action. It is dangerous for any man to attribute motives, lest he fall under the condemnation of "bearing false witness against his neighbor." In relation to myself I desire to say but little. I prefer to be judged by my actions. *It is not true* that I availed myself of the benefits of the act of Congress to which you refer by seeking a high command under it. I offered service and was accepted as captain of my company, without any pledge or understanding, directly or indirectly, that I was to have any other commission. My present office of Colonel of this regiment has been conferred upon me through the voluntary confidence of the President, and through the wish, as I have reason to believe, of every officer and private under my command. I have desired no office, prefering, for many reasons, to remain at the head of my company, between which and myself there has existed a deep-seated attachment, and it was only by their consent that I agreed to command the regiment. My reasons for entering the service are very simple. I had labored as much as any man in Georgia to effect the secession of the State; I had pledged myself to meet all the consequences of secession. I am bound, therefore, in honor, and still more strongly by duty, to be among the foremost in accepting the bloody consequences which seem to threaten us. My life can be as well spared as any other man's, and I am willing and ready to devote it. You taunt me with deserting my home and the defence of my fireside "to serve the common cause in a more pleasant summer climate." I wish you were here to witness the realities of this service you deem so pleasant. It would cure you, I think, of some of your malicious propensities. You taunt me with having imposed upon others the duty of defending the post which I have deserted, and yet when you penned this you knew that you had steadily refused to call the volunteer troops of Savannah into service of any kind, and that you had called "many of our bravest young men from other parts of the State to fill our places" and defend our homes, while we were permitted to rest in inglorious ease. The volunteer troops of Savannah are now in service, not through *you*, but by the direct order of the Commander-in-chief of the Confederate forces. All that you say upon this subject is Jesuitical, designed to subserve a purpose rather than narrate the truth. I have the same right to judge that you have as to the probability of an attack upon Savannah. There is scarcely a seaboard city along the Atlantic coast that has not its representatives here in Virginia. Why should Savannah be an exception? Surely one company could be spared, at least, to show that her heart beat true to the common cause, and that her youth were ready to court danger upon the very frontiers of the war. Such a spirit is not what you have characterized it. It is probably above your comprehension, but the generous and noble-hearted of my native State will know how to appreciate it.

And now as to my arms. I did not ask you to arm and equip me. I had already received from the late government of the United States, through you, arms and equipments which cost the State of Georgia nothing. They were delivered to me and you took my bond for their safe keeping, unless destroyed in the *public service.* You have threatened me with the penalty of that bond. Take it if you can get it. That is your remedy. If I have been wrong in taking the arms away from Georgia, I am a trespasser and of course responsible. I think the power you claim to disarm companies once armed and under bonds, at your will, is, to say the least of it, doubtful. As I have already said, in a former letter, I would not make this issue if I could find any way to avoid it. I would rather yield than have a controversy with any man where the public interests are involved. But situated as I was, I prefer disobedience, if you please, rather than to jeopard the honor and safety of one hundred men confided to my care. You seem to think I am arrogant in claiming our humble share in representing the State of Georgia on this field of action. You say that you are not aware of the State authority by which I am called to represent the State of Georgia in Virginia. You make here again, your common error, of supposing that *you are the State of Georgia,*—a mistake in which I do not participate. You will not be permitted to alienate from us the esteem and affection of those we leave behind, and whom we love so dearly. I am sorry that you have undertaken so ungracious a task.

You say "that at present I am beyond the reach of State authority, and State lines, so far as I am concerned, are obliterated. How long this may remain so," you say, "depends upon the developments of the future." I trust, if God spares my life, I shall set foot again upon the soil of Georgia, and be well assured that I no more fear to meet my enemies at home than I now do to meet the enemies of my country abroad.

With due respect. I have the honor to be, your most obedient

FRANCIS S. BARTOW.

Soon after his arrival in Virginia he was appointed Colonel of the 8th Georgia regiment, and at the first battle of Manassas he was commanding a brigade composed of the 7th, 8th, 9th, and 11th Georgia, and the 1st Kentucky regiments. During the engagement only the 7th and 8th Georgia regiments were engaged. During the forepart of the battle his command suffered heavily, and at noon, when it became necessary for the left of our army to fall back to its original position, occupied early in the morning, his regiments also retired. During this movement General Bartow rode up to General Beauregard, the general commanding, and said: "What shall now be done? Tell me, and if human efforts can avail, I will do it." General Beauregard, pointing to a battery at the Stone Bridge, replied: "That battery should be silenced." Seizing the standard of the 7th Georgia regiment, and calling upon the remnants of his command to follow him, he led the van in the charge. A ball wounded him slightly and killed his horse under him. Still grasping the standard, and rising again, he mounted another horse, and waving his cap around his head, cheered his troops to come on. They followed. Another ball pierced his heart and he fell to the ground, exclaiming to those who gathered around him, "THEY HAVE KILLED ME, BUT NEVER GIVE UP THE FIELD," and expired. His dying injunction was obeyed. His command proceeded on the charge and silenced the battery under the protection of which the enemy had hurled the missile of death into the heart of one whose fall plunged a struggling nation into mourning.

The deceased was as marked in character as distinguished for talent. He was ardent in friendships—sincere and ingenious in his professions—of a lofty sense of honor—chivalric in the tone of his sentiments—patriotic in his ambition—brave by nature and constitution—generous in his impulses—most zealous in his devotion to truth—deeply imbued with the religious sentiment and cherished a reverential regard for all of the institutions of religion. His style of oratory was bold, earnest, and impassioned. As a criminal advocate, his eloquence was of a high, thrilling order; and his efforts in important criminal trials established for him a fame which will live with the memory of his beloved and honored name. He was astute as a lawyer and profound in his legal attainments. His literary attainments were varied and extensive, while his familiarity with the classics was intimate. His perception and love for the beautiful in art and nature were keen and warm—his imagination was rich and glowing, and his thoughts were always fervid.

In July, 1861, Hon. T. R. R. Cobb, before the Congress of the Confederate States of America, in session in Richmond, Virginia, pronounced an eloquent eulogy upon General Bartow, after which the following resolutions were offered and unanimously adopted:

Resolved, That Congress has heard with unfeigned sorrow of the death of the Honorable Francis S. Bartow, one of the delegates from the State of Georgia; that the natural exultation for a glorious victory achieved by our arms is checked by the heavy loss sustained by the Confederacy in the death of one of her most efficient counsellors; and that, as his colleagues, we feel a peculiar loss to ourselves, in one who had won our esteem and gained our affection.

Resolved, That with pleasure we record our admiration of his heroic defence on the field of battle of the action of Congress in which he participated so largely, and find some consolation for his death in the conviction that his noble self-sacrifice will serve to establish the work which he so boldly aided to begin.

Resolved, That we appreciate the loss which Georgia, his native State, has sustained in the death of one of her noblest sons, and that we tender to the bereaved family the sympathy of hearts, to some extent, stricken by the same blow which has crushed their own.

Resolved, That in testimony of our respect for his memory, the Congress do now adjourn.

The Chatham Artillery was organized on the 1st of May, 1786, and was included in the surrender of the Confederate troops by General Joseph E. Johnston. The battery served at Fort Pulaski and other points around Savannah; at Olustee; at Secessionville, Battery Wagner, and other points around Charleston; and with the Western army until its surrender. The guns of the battery were surrendered on the seventy-ninth anniversary of the organization. The battery at that time consisted of four twelve-pounder Napoleon guns, two of which were Federal guns, captured at the battle of Olustee and given to the battery by the General commanding in token of his appreciation of the distinguished services and gallant conduct of its members during that battle. The following were officers of the battery at various periods from the commencement to the close of the war: Captain Joseph S. Claghorn (promoted to colonel), Lieutenants C. C. Jones (promoted to lieutenant-colonel), Julian Hartridge (elected member of the Confederate Congress), William M. Davidson (promoted to captain), B. S. Sanchez, T. A. Askew, John F. Wheaton (promoted to captain of the battery early in the war and remained in command until the close), George A. Whitehead, S. B. Palmer and George N. Hendry.

The Georgia Hussars were organized in 1796, and went into service at the commencement of the war, and in September, 1861, succeeded in obtaining permission to go to Virginia, and served throughout the war with the army of Northern Virginia. Captain J. F. Waring, the captain at the time of entering service, was promoted to colonel of the Jeff. Davis Legion, and Lieutenant David Waldhauer was promoted to captain; Lieutenant W. W. Gordon was promoted to captain on General Mercer's staff; and A. McC. Duncan was promoted to 1st lieutenant, and J. L. McTurner and Robert Saussey elected lieutenants. The second company (known as company B) was organized in November, 1861, under Captain W. H. Wiltberger (promoted to major of the 5th Georgia Cavalry), Lieutenants R. J. Davant (promoted to lieutenant-colonel of the same regiment), M. E. Williams, and F. Williams. In 1862 the company was reorganized under Captain Wiltberger, Lieutenants James A. Zittrouer, E. P. Hill, and Phillip Yonge. Lieutenant Hill resigned, and Fred. H. Blois was elected lieutenant. At the promotion of Captain Wiltberger, Lieutenant Zittrouer became captain. The lieutenants were advanced a grade and John H. Ashe was elected lieutenant. The company was with the 5th Georgia Cavalry, and served around Savannah, on the South Carolina coast, in Florida, and with the Western army.

The Savannah Volunteer Guards were organized in 1802, and until the commencement of the late war were commanded by Captains John Cumming, M. D., J. Marshall, F. Fell, Edward F. Tattnall, Joseph W. Jackson, William Robertson, Cosmo P. Richardsone, M. D., James P. Screven, and John Screven—the latter-named officer being in command of the company when it aided in seizing Fort Pulaski on the 3d of January, 1861. The lieutenants then were: A. C. Davenport, W. S. Basinger, and G. C. Rice. Early in 1861, so great was the number of volunteers to the company, it became necessary to organize another, the two being respectively known as companies A and B. The officers of company A were: Captain John Screven, Lieutenants W. S. Basinger, G. C. Rice, and J. C. Habersham; and Captain A. C. Davenport, Lieutenants G. W. Stiles, M. H. Hopkins, and Thomas F. Screven officers of company B. In March, 1862, the corps, numbering three companies, was mustered into service as a battalion for the war. Captain John Screven became Major of the battalion, the companies being officered as follows: Company A, Captain W. S. Basinger, Lieutenants T. F. Screven, William H. King, and Fred.

Tupper. Company B, Captain George W. Stiles, Lieutenants E. Padelford, jr., E. A. Castellaw, and George D. Smith. Company C, Captain G. C. Rice, Lieutenants G. M. Turner, John R. Dillon, and E. Blois. Late in 1862 Major Screven resigned (afterward appointed lieutenant-colonel of local battalion) and Captain Basinger succeeded to the command of the battalion. The Lieutenants in company A were advanced a grade and Sergeant P. N. Raynal elected lieutenant. Lieutenant Padelford, of company B, died in June, 1863, and Sergeant W. E. Gue was elected a lieutenant, the other lieutenants having been advanced a grade. In December, 1863, Lieutenant Castellaw, of company B, resigned; the other lieutenants were advanced a grade and Sergeant W. D. Grant was elected lieutenant. The battalion officers were: Major W. S. Basinger, Adjutant E. P. Starr, Captain R. H. Footman, A. Q. M., George W. Coxwell, Surgeon. The battalion was known as the 18th Georgia Battalion, and served around Savannah and around Charleston, participating in the defence of Battery Wagner. In May, 1864, the battalion was ordered to Virginia, and participated in the last battles of the Army of Northern Virginia, being badly cut up at Sailor's Creek, a few days before the surrender of General Lee.

The Republican Blues were organized in 1808, and served in the late war under Captain John W. Anderson, who resigned and was succeeded by George W. Anderson (afterward promoted to Major in the regular army), Lieutenants George A. Nicoll, W. D. Dixon, T. C. Elkins, F. Willis, and J. M. Theus. Lieutenant Nicoll was promoted to Captain of the Emmett Rifles and Lieutenant Dixon became captain of the Blues. This company served at Fort McAllister and other points around Savannah, and with the Western army, being connected with the 1st Georgia regiment.

The Phœnix Riflemen were organized on the 1st of May, 1830, and went into service at the commencement of the war under Captain George A. Gordon (promoted to colonel of the 63d Georgia regiment), Lieutenants George R. Black (promoted to lieutenant-colonel of the same regiment), George W. Lamar (promoted to the rank of captain), Spaulding McIntosh, George R. Giles (promoted to major of the 63d Georgia regiment). The ranks of the company were constantly increased, which necessitated the forming of two other companies. The three companies were organized into a battalion, and afterward, with additional companies, organized into a regiment, known as the 63d Georgia. The three companies served around Savannah and in the Western army, under Captain James T. Buckner, Lieutenants William Lyons, William E. Readick, James Geary, and G. A. Bailey, of the first company; Captain John H. Lopez, Lieutenants L. T. Turner, John Smith, and Eldred Gefckin, of the second company; Captain William Dixon, Lieutenants Charles Law and Joseph Keiffer, of the third company.

The Irish Jasper Greens were organized on the 22d of February, 1843, and served in the Mexican war. During the late war they were officered by Captain John Flannery, Lieutenants Thomas Mahoney, John Greene, and Edmund Flaherty. The ranks of the company were increased above the number allowed, and on the 4th of February, 1862, company B was organized under Captain David O'Connor, Lieutenants James Dooner, John Deacy, Peter Reiley, Michael Goodwin, and Wm. H. Dooner. Captain O'Connor died during service and Lieutenant James Dooner became captain. Both companies were in the 1st Georgia regiment, and shared its fortunes while around Savannah and with the Western army.

The German Volunteers were organized on the 22d of February, 1846, and went into service under Captain John H. Stegin, Lieutenants A. Basler, C. Werner, and C. H. A. Umbach. The company was captured at Fort Pulaski, and, when exchanged, reorganized under Captain C. Werner, Lieutenants C. H. A. Umbach, I. Fleck, and I. Wolber. Captain Werner was killed and Lieutenant Umbach became captain; the other officers were promoted, and George Murkins became a lieutenant. This company served around Savannah, at Battery Wagner, and with the Western army, forming a part of the 1st Georgia regiment.

The DeKalb Riflemen were organized in 1850, and went into service under the following officers: Captain P. Wetter, Lieutenants A. L. Hartridge, B. H. Hardee, and Henry Herman. The company was reorganized in 1862, and Lieutenant Hartridge was promoted to captain. The other lieutenants were advanced a grade and T. S. Wayne elected a lieutenant. Captain Hartridge was promoted to Major of Artillery, and Lieutenant Hardee became captain and Robert Wayne was elected a lieutenant. The company served along the coast, and in 1863 was placed in the Georgia Sharpshooters battalion, and participated in the various battles of the army of the West.

The Oglethorpe Light Infantry were organized on the 8th of January, 1856, the first captain being John N. Lewis. Francis S. Bartow was elected captain in 1857, and was in command when the company assisted in seizing Fort Pulaski on the 3d of January, 1861. The company left for Virginia on the 21st of May, 1861, having been reorganized previous to starting. The lieutenants then were: J. J. West, Hamilton Couper, and A. F. Butler. Captain Bartow was promoted to brigadier-general and killed at Manassas. Lieutenant West became captain, but resigned shortly afterward, and Lieutenant Couper was elected captain. Captain Couper died in 1862, and Lieutenant Butler succeeded to the captaincy, remaining in that position until the surrender of the company at Appomattox Courthouse, Virginia. The lieutenants during service were: J. L. Holcombe (promoted to major and killed at Jonesboro), Fred. Bliss, S. W. Branch, P. B. Holmes, E. Starke Law. This company was the first company in the South to offer its services for the war, and served in all the battles of the army of Northern Virginia, and was with Longstreet's corps when it made its celebrated circuit of the Confederacy. It formed part of the 8th Georgia regiment, which was so highly complimented by General Beauregard for its bravery during the first battle of Manassas. Previous to the company's departure for Virginia, in 1861, the number of volunteers had increased its ranks beyond the maximum number, and another company, known as the Oglethorpe Light Infantry, company B, was organized under Captain F. W. Sims, Lieutenants Henry C. Freeman, Benjamin T. Cole, and James Lachlison. The company was captured at Fort Pulaski, and, on being exchanged, reorganized and served under Captain James Lachlison, jr., Lieutenants H. A. Elkins, Joshua C. Bruyn, and James Simmons. Captain Sims, shortly after his exchange, was promoted to lieutenant-colonel and assigned to duty in Richmond, Va. This company formed part of the 1st Georgia regiment, and participated with it in the various battles around Charleston and those fought by the army of the West.

The 1st Georgia regiment was composed of the old volunteer companies of Savannah, but was reorganized after hostilities commenced, with the following companies composing it: Republican Blues, Irish Jasper Greens (first and second companies), German Volunteers, Oglethorpe Light Infantry (company B), Washington Volunteers, Tatnall Guards, Coast Rifles, City Light Guard, and Irish Volunteers. The officers of the regiment were: Colonel Charles H. Olmstead, Lieutenant-Colonel W. S. Rockwell, who resigned and Major Martin J. Ford became lieutenant-colonel, Major John Foley, who resigned and Captain S. Yates Levy was appointed major; and Adjutant M. H. Hopkins. The regiment, or a portion of it, was at Fort Pulaski when it was besieged; also at Battery Wagner, with the army of the West, and at Fort McAllister.

The City Light Guards were organized on the 4th of March, 1861, and served under the following officers: Captain S. Yates Levy, Lieutenants Robert H. Elliott, George C. Nichols, C. M. Cunningham, Joseph P. White, John J. Tidwell, and Robert H. Lewis. After the promotion of Captain Levy to major, Lieutenant Cunningham became captain.

The Washington Volunteers were organized in August, 1861, under Captain John McMahon, Lieutenants Francis P. Blair, C. D. Rogers, J. C. Rowland, and A. G. McArthur. The company was captured at Fort Pulaski, and when exchanged, reorganized under Captain John Cooper, Lieutenants J. C. Rowland, A. G. McArthur, and T. C. Bates.

The Tattnall Guards were organized, shortly after the commencement of hostilities, under Captain A. C. Davenport, Lieutenants B. H. Cole, John D. Hopkins, and Cyrus B. Carter.

The Irish Volunteers were organized early in 1861 (for six months), under Captain Jacob B. Read, Lieutenants Henry Williams, and A. J. J. Blois. At the expiration of this period the company was disbanded. Previous to this another company, under the same name and the following officers, was organized, and many of the members of the old company joined it: Captain John F. O'Neal, Lieutenants Robert Denver and Henry O'Neal.

The Coast Rifles were organized early in 1861, under Captain Screven Turner, Lieutenants Thaddeus Fisher, E. A. Castellaw, John Coburn, and Charles Webster. Captain Turner was killed, and Lieutenant Fisher became captain.

The Emmett Rifles were organized in August, 1861, under the following officers: Captain A. Bonaud (afterward organized a battalion, of which he became major), Lieutenants William E. Long (afterward promoted to captain, A. Q. M.), W. S. Rockwell, and George Dickerson. At the reorganization, in 1862, George A. Nicoll was elected captain. Lieutenant Rockwell retained his position, and Edgar M. McDonnell was elected lieutenant. The company served along the coast, and participated in the numerous engagements at Fort McAllister, and was there captured.

The Savannah Cadets were organized on the 17th of May, 1816, and served along the coast of Georgia and South Carolina until April, 1864, when they were ordered to the Western army, and shared the fortunes of that army until its surrender, under Captain Walter S. Chisholm (who resigned in 1863 to accept the judgeship of the City Court), Lieutenants John W. Anderson (promoted to captain after Captain Chisholm resigned), H. M. Branch, C. C. Hunter and P. R. Falligant.

The Oglethorpe Siege Artillery was organized early in 1862, and served in the batteries around Savannah and Charleston, and in the Western army after the evacuation of Savannah, under Captain John Lama, Lieutenants Algernon Hartridge, Milton C. Wade, R. R. Richards, and Alexander Campbell.

The Blue Cap Cavalry was organized in March, 1861, and served in Georgia, Florida, North Carolina, South Carolina, Tennessee, and Virginia, under Captain Isaac M. Marsh, Lieutenants W. F. Walton, Samuel Lewis, and John R. Freyer.

The Mitchell Volunteer Guards were organized on the 4th of March, 1862, and served around Savannah and Charleston, and in the Western army, under Captain M. J. Doyle (who resigned and was succeeded by Lieutenant B. Connor), Lieutenants P. W. Doyle, and John Joseph Purtell.

The Montgomery Guards were organized on the 20th of August, 1861, under Captain L. J. Guilmartin, Lieutenants John J. Symons, Christopher Hussey, and Christopher Murphy. The company was captured at Fort Pulaski, and when exchanged reorganized, electing Lieutenant Christopher Hussey captain, and Christopher Murphy, J. J. Symons, and W. V. Apperson lieutenants. The company served around Savannah and in the Western army. Captain Hussey died just before General Joseph E. Johnston's surrender, and Lieutenant Murphy was promoted to captain.

The Savannah Artillery was organized in 1860, under Captain John B. Gallie (promoted to major and killed at Fort McAllister). George L. Cope became captain, and B. Whitehead, E. Knapp, and C. W. Holst lieutenants. The company served around Savannah until 1862, when it was disbanded, and the members volunteered in other companies.

SAVANNAH'S ROLL OF HONOR.

Those marked thus * were killed; those marked † died in service or since the war; and those marked ‡ were wounded.

MAJOR-GENERALS

J. F. Gilmer, Geo. P. Harrison, Commodore J. Tatnall.

BRIGADIER-GENERALS

R. H. Anderson, Isaac W. Avery, Ed. C. Anderson, Francis S. Bartow,* J. S. Bowen,* William R. Boggs, Henry R. Jackson, W. W. Kirkland, A. R. Lawton,‡ H. W. Mercer, G. Moxley Sorrell.

COLONELS

Edward C. Anderson, Joseph S. Claghorn, Winder P. Johnson, George A. Gordon, Charles A. L. Lamar,* J. M. Millen,* Charles H. Olmstead, F. W. Simms, W. R. Symons, W. T. Thompson, J. F. Waring,‡ W. M. Wadley, Charlton H. Way, R. A. Wayne, Aaron Wilbur.

LIEUTENANT-COLONELS

George R. Black, Richard J. Davant, Jr., Martin J. Ford, B. B. Ferrill, C. C. Jones, W. R. Pritchard, W. S. Rockwell, John Screven.

MAJORS

George W. Anderson, W. S. Basinger,‡ P. H. Behn, T. D. Bertody, A. Bonaud. Henry Bryan, John Cunningham, H. N. Davenport, R. W. B. Elliott, John Foley, T. J. Charlton, John M. Guerard, Geo. R. Giles,‡ Jno. B. Gallie,* E. L. Holcombe, A. L. Hartridge, J. L. Holcombe,* Charles S. Hardee, B. W. Hardee, J. C. Habersham, J. M, Johnston, W. S. Lawton, S. Yates Levy, J. C. Le Hardy, McPherson B. Millen, D. H. Morrisson, J. T. McFarland, J. B. Read, James T. Stewart, W. F. Shellman, J. G. Thomas, Joseph C. Thompson,‡ J. J. Waring, W. D. Waples, W. H. Wiltberger, J. S. Williams.

CAPTAINS

John W. Anderson,† John W. Anderson, Jr., R. F. Aiken, James T. Buckner, A. F. Butler,‡ W. H. Burroughs, Jr., N. B. Brown, J. McP. Berrien,‡ A. Basler, George S. Barthelmess, De Witt C. Bruyn, George W. Coxwell, T. M. Cunningham, C. M. Cunningham, S. M. Colding, John Cooper, Walter S. Chisolm, B. Connor, George L. Cope, Hamilton Couper,† E. Chevis,* H. C. Cunningham, J. S. Campfield, William M. Davidson, J. H. Demund, H. W. Denslow, A. C. Davenport, William Dixon, William D. Dixon, James Dooner, Archibald C. Davenport, George Dickerson, M. J. Doyle, E. W. Drummond, William Duncan, Robert

Erwin, W. H. Elliott, R. H. Footman, John Flannery, Thaddeus Fisher, F. L. Gue, W. W. Gordon, L. J. Guilmartin, E. L. Guerard, James B. Grant,† C. R. Goodwin, Thomas B. Gowen, B. H. Hardee, Christopher Hussey,† W. F. Holland, J. D. Hopkins, R. B. Harris, W. D. Harden, C. C. Hardwicke, Jno. Howard, Jno. R. Johnson, J. S. Kennard, Geo. W. Lamar, Jno. H. Lopez,‡ Jas. Lachlison, Jr.,‡ Wm. E. Long, W. F. Law, G. B. Lamar, T. B. Lamar, E. P. Lawton,* Jno. Lama, R. E. Lester, J. M. B. Lovell, Spaulding McIntosh, John McMahon, I. M. Marsh, Christopher Murphy, J. W. McAlpin, George A. Mercer, Robert P. Myers, George A. Nicoll, R. J. Nunn, John F. O'Neal, David O'Connor,† D. G. Purse, William H. Patterson,‡ G. C. Rice,* A. Richardson, A. M. Richards, T. F. Screven, George W. Stiles, John H. Stegin, C. A. Stiles, H. H. Scranton,† F. C. Sollee, A. C. Sorrell, Robert Stiles, John W. Sutlive, Screven Turner,* J. S. Turner,* J. H. Thomas, H. A. Umbach,‡ John F. Wheaton, C. H. Wylly, W. L. Walthour, C. J. White, R. D. Walker, David Waldhauer,‡ C. Werner,* P. Wetter, J. J. West, R. Habersham Wylly.

LIEUTENANTS

T. A. Askew, John H. Ashe, A. G. McArthur, W. V. Apperson, Ed. M. Anderson. Frederick H. Blois, E. Blois,* G. A. Bailey, A. Basler, Joshua C. Bruyn, Francis P. Blair, T. C. Bates, A. J. J. Blois, H. M. Branch,‡ Fred Bliss,* S. M. Branch,‡ L. C. Berrien, Jno. S. Branch,* John Bilbo, Sam'l P. Bell, Henry Butler, Jno. S. Butler, Edward A. Castellaw,‡ Benjamin T. Cole, B. H. Cole, Cyrus B. Carter,* John Coburn, H. A. Crane, A. T. Cunningham, C. M. Cunningham, John R. Dillon,‡ John Deacey, W. H. Dooner, Robert Denver, P. W. Doyle, George W. Dickerson, R. M. Demere, G. Darling, T. C. Elkins, H. A. Elkins,‡ Robert H. Elliott, Paul Elkins, Edmund Flaherty, I. Fleck, Henry C. Freeman,‡ P. R. Falligant,‡ John R. Freyer, J. M. Fleming,* Robert Falligant, C. G. Falligant, W. E. Gue, W. D. Grant,† James W. Geary, Eldred Gefckin, John Greene, Michael Goodwin, W. E. Guerard, A. H. Gordon, W. R. Gignilliatt, Joseph H. Gnann,* Robert Grant,† William T. Gibson, G. P. Goodwin, Julian Hartridge, Algernon Hartridge, E. P. Hill, M. H. Hopkins, John D. Hopkins, Henry Herman,* C. C. Hunter,‡ C. W. Holst, P. B. Holmes,* F. A. Habersham,* J. T. Howard, James Hunter,‡ Jr., J. L. Hammond, George N. Hendry, James Hunter, G. H. Johnston, W. H. King,* Joseph Keiffer,* E. Knapp, William Lyons, Charles Law,‡ Robert H. Lewis,‡ Samuel Lewis, E. Starke Law,‡ A. B. Luce, John A. Lewis, A. McC. Duncan, Thomas Mahoney, George Murkins, Edgar N. McDonnell, F. J. McCall, Edward Manes, M. Molina,* John L. Martin, T. A. Maddox, J. B. McIntosh, John Mahoney, L. Y. Mallory, George C. Nichols, Henry O'Neal,* S. P. Norris, E. F. Neufville, John Oliver, S. B. Palmer, E. Padelford, Jr.,† John J. Purtell,† C. A. Patillo,† George T. Patten, Charles T. Preston, P. N. Raynal, W. E. Readick,* Peter Reily, C. D. Rogers, J. C. Roland, W. S. Rockwell, J. A. Rahn, William Rogers, C. B. Richardson, J. C. Roland, W. A. Russell, R. R. Richards, B. S. Sanchez,* Robert Saussy, George D. Smith,† E. P. Starr,‡ John Smith,† James Simmons, H. B. Saddler, W. P. Schrom, G. P. Screven, H. R. Symons, J. L. McTurner, Fred. Tupper,† G. M. Turner,* L. T. Turner,‡ J. M. Theus,‡ J. J. Tidwell, George A. Whitehead, M. E. Williams, F. Williams, F. Willis, I. Wolber, Joseph P. White, Henry Williams, Charles Webster, Thomas S. Wayne, Robert Wayne,‡ W. F. Walton, B. Whitehead, A. A. Ward,* Michael Walsh, H. K. Washburne, H. Way, Milton C. Wade, Philip Yonge.

PRIVATES

I. Ames,† J. H. Austin, H. Atkinson, J. M. Abrahams,† R. E. Allen, W. C. Avery, B. Abney,* J. G. Ardis, L. B. Andrew, J. J. Abrams, A. Alleoud, A. S. Achord, James L. Agnew, G. S. Appleton, J. H. Ashe, R. W. Adams, J. T. Austin, D. E. Ardis, James Aaron, J. O. Andrews, C. Y. Anderson, George Atchison, Robert Andrews, Joseph Adams, W. L. B. Aikens, William Allen, J. Abramscyk, James M. Ashfield,† William Ashfield, John D. Audas, George R. Anderson,† William Anderson, D. O. Avery,* R. Attaway, D. R. Adams, W. Adams, A. J. Adams, I. T. Adams, William Allison, George Archibald, G. H. Angill, David A. Adams, George F. Allen, L. Aikens, W. Andrews.

W. T. Borchert,† J. A. Brown, Samuel Brown,‡ George M. Barnes,† Robert Bren, L. Bevill,† E. J. Bourquin,† Thaddeus W. Bennett, G. D. Baker,† W. H. Bourne,‡ Berry Bradford, W. B. Bradford,‡ W. H. Bird, Wm. R. Boyd, C. F. Borchert, S. H. Baldie,* W. H. Bennett, E. B. Barnwell,* W. H. Barton, Robert Q. Baker,‡ I. H. Bogart, M. B. Boston,* Willis A. Burney,‡ George M. Butler,* Jno. A. Belvin,‡ DeWitt C. Bacon, F. W. Baily,† W. S. Bogart, Lewis Bliss, John Bilbo, Alfred Bliss,† Osceola Butler, R. F. Baker, M. O'Byrne, W. C. Bishop, A. M. Bowen, J. S. Bayard, J. H. Bowman, M. Burns, W. E. Q. Baker, Richard Broderick, Alfred Bishop, A. Boulineau, J. G. Barnwell, M. J. Bayard, C. J. Barrie, J. H. Butler,† W. J. Bee, M. A. Barrie, L. E. Barrie,* J. C. Bryan,† Hugh Bryan, Gideon Bliss,† J. W. Burroughs, W. H. Bradley, Thos. Byrns, T. P. Bond, M. T. Bruner, W. C. Bennett,* C. Barnwell, H. Baars,‡ James Bryan,* J. J. Butler,† James Belote,‡ Henry Bennett, H. H. Black, B. Brady, H. M. Bryan, Isaac Brunner, David Bell, T. J. Bulloch, A. O. Bowie,* P. N. Box, A. M. Barber, Eugene Bee, E. H. Bacon, H. G. Black, J. B. Bennett, John'Blackie, C. W. Brunner, H. F. Bruen,† A. E. W. Barclay, J. Borrel, O. T. Bacon, H. N. Bryan, W. J. Bessent, A. S. Bacon, J. H. Barton, L. E. Baly, C. W. Bruen, J. T. Baker, R. J. R. Bee, B. Brunner, Geo. R. Black, S. J. M. Baker, Henry Bryan, A. M. Barbee, C. J. Bartlett, John Barrie, J. J. Butler,† J. A. Baker,† E. H. Bacon, A. Barrie, J. S. Bryan, W. H. Bulloch, T. R. Brannon, F. Bacchus, J. O. Bryin, C. Brukman,* W. Brewer, F. Bierhalter, W. Brooks, J. W. Booth,‡ D. Brewer, D. Browen, L. Brown,‡ C. Beckton,‡ R. A. F. Blakeley,‡ H. Black, R. Barrett, W. Backley,‡ A. Beyard, H. Bridie,† T. A. Batton, W. Baxter, J. Bryant,‡ J. E. Beasley, W. Beasley, H. Bogardus, W. G. Bruce,* J. Brady, J. Bessent, T. Bennett, T. Blessing, W. W. Bradley,† F. S. Battley,‡ J. R. Browne, J. M. Boyd, A. M. Buford, G. A. Bailie, T. S. Bird, L. Burroughs, S. R. Banks, H. O. Best, J. W. Bieze, T. J. Bransby, C. P. Burkhalter, W. Best, L. A. Butts, James D. Bell, William H. Bell, William Best, L. A. Butts,, J. C. Browning.‡ J. W. Bailey,| C. B. Browning, J. Brown, P. C. Brown, I. Bell, Wm. Burns, P. Burket, A. P. Boggs, G. A. Blount, G. Burns, S. H. Bowman, John W. Baley, Charles H. Baker, Stephen J. Baker, J. J. Boyd, R. E. Brantly, David H. Bailey, John Barrie, E. W. Brown, H. L. Benning, George W. Blount, George W. Brownell, Thomas Blitch, William C. Bradley, J. J. Barron,‡ Henry J. Byrd, L. Bragg,‡ D. J. Bryant, R. J. G. Blake, William Bray, I. M. Beck, John Brein,‡ B. Bryant, Charles Berry, Mark Breen, James Brannon, James Bray, Ed. Brady, John Blessing, Michael Black, T. Berryhill, Patrick Barrett, George W. Berry, H. F. Beach, William Box, W. W. Brown, M. Bozman, Henry C. Bradley, Robert A. Beasley, Ed. W. Barnwell, William Burnham, William Black, Joseph P. Bell, Robert Barnwell, Lawrence C. Butler, William M. Butler, John Brady,

J. A. Bessinger, Peter Burket, S. S. Bessinger,‡ J. E. Beasley, C. A. Barron, J. R. B. Baker, Charles Blaque,† G. F. Basefield, H. Bingham,‡ John Baker,‡ John Berkley, M. Buchanon, John Brantley, Wm. Butler, Henry Bennar, Richard Burke,‡ Michael Barrett,† Thomas Brennan, John Brasnahan, James Brennan, James Bent,‡ William Burns, Michael Bryan, G. Baukman, James Barbour,‡ Charles F. Blancho, Charles R. Badger, Wm. J. Baillie,‡ Wm. Barbour,‡ B. B. Baillie, M. Bishop, James Bishop, John A. Baynes, Wm. H. Bonner,‡ Thos. H. Butler, Wm. Bell, Thos. B. Bond, R. F. W. Burroughs,† Franklin Bird,† Barry Byrd,† Henry E. Ball, J. W. Biggs, Thomas Ballantyne, W. Baynard,* J. A. Boughan, John A. Britton,‡ John Burnett, George W. Bockley,† F. Brodbacker (killed by negroes, Dec. 1868, while on patrol duty), L. Brum, J. F. Butler,‡ Dominique Brown,‡ John T. Blatz, H. Bergner, Dennis Boyle.†

William C. Crawford, Harry A. Carter,† J. J. Crumpler,† Thomas Cuddigan,† Z. Castleberry, W. H. Crane,* I. E. Carolan,* I. B. Chisholm, R. H. Cole,‡ William Combs,* A. H. Charlton, Charles Cevor, W. B. Corey, R. A. Crawford, Charles Cannon,† H. R. Christian, Daniel Callahan, James Coleman, James Cooper, Wm. Craven, John Cheisman, Pat. Cashin, W. J. Cash,† J. M. Cole, W. R. Cooke, G. B. Clarke, N. Corbin, J. Cooner, A. H. Champion, J. B. Crabtree, R. M. Charlton,† L. Connell,‡ Isaac Cohen, George A. Cuyler,† C. C. Cushing, D. J. Craft, J. M. Carrol,† A. W. Clarke, E. Copeland,† John Chipman, C. Clarke, H. Crook,* J. J. Cornell, S. Coalson, J. Carmody,† H. M. Comstock,† P. Cooney, J. Carroll, B. Coldman, T. J. Crotty, A. Cowper, M. S. Cohen, G. S. H. Clarke, J. G. Cornell, J. Conlan,* John Cooper, J. S. Caruthers, James Chaplin, Ed. Cooper, John Calder, Robert Cessor, John Cooper, W. T. Coleman, A. J. Coleman, Thomas Cobb, Geo. Clark, Barnet Carr, Maurice Crowley, Thos. Carlin, James Clancey, Wm. Condon, Patrick Curran, Stephen Clark, E. W. Cribb, Nathan Childre, Richard Crotty, Andrew Collins, E. J. Connell, George Cambeff, F. B. Colson, John Curren, John G. Cushing, John W. Counts, M. Cohen, Wm. H. Cardwell, James Coil, Edward F. Costigan, Martin Connor,* J. A. Calloway, A. R. Cullens, George Cordes, Theodore Carnis, Washington Cole, Thomas B. Clare, D. L. Cole, Thomas Carrolan, F. B. Cocke,† James C. Chisolm, A. Chisolm, P. I. Creagan, Mathew Clancey, L. Callahan, Nicholas Cullen,† P. Campbell,† J. Crinmon, Michael Cusick, Garrett Coltor, P. Connahan, P. Condon,† Michael Cleary, Thomas Conghlin,† Luke Carson, Cornelius Cronin, John Coleman, James Crotty, Thomas Carroll, Richard Crotty, P. Cullen, Michael Cumins, Michael Cash, Jeremiah Crowley, John Cooney, Thomas Cooney, Michael Copps, William J. Cook, DeWitt C. Cook, Isaac S. Cohen, P. G. Cope,‡ Joseph J. Cooper, Ed. Clifford, Morris Cohen, Pat. Carlis, L. J. Connell, John W. Calloway,† Jos. J. Clarke, Hardy Cook, J. C. Connell, L. H. Clemens,‡ A. J. Campbell,† Robert Campbell,† T. B. Chisolm, I. W. C. Clarke, Alfred Cuthbert, Michael Clarke, C. N. Clemens,† Jacob Clemens, J. W. Crew,‡ L. Calahan,† L. Cason,† M. J. Cox,† L. Cox,† John Carter,† R. Carson, C. Christie,‡ C. Campbell, David Carter, R. Cercopaly, W. Curry, W. A. Conery, J. D. Claherty, James Cauffield, Allen Cullen, T. H. Courter, G. H. Cox, J. W. Connor, G. W. Clarke, W. H. Cooper, J. H. Cullen, Floyd Crockett, G. Carswell, E. Clarke, Benj. Carter,* Arthur Connoway, James L. Crosby, George Cash,* John Crosby, D. Wiley Carter, W. W. Connor, John B. Connor,† R. A. Crawford, Milton Creighton, R. Carroll, A. Cowan,† L. M. Cowan, W. W. Cheever, F. B. Cleary, F. A. Canuet, G. R. Clarke, C. P. Carey, W. G. Cooper.

N. J. Darrell, M. Davis,* Thomas Devane, Alfred Davis, B. Dunovan,‡ S. M.

Dasher,* W. B. Dasher,‡ Joseph O. Davis,‡ Henry L. Davis,‡ George Dell, O. Dauvergne,‡ J. H. Demund, J. G. Deitz, Jacob F. Doe,† H. B. Dumas, Thomas Dunn, John Dreesen, G. E. Dixon, J. M. Davis,† R. L. Dixon, H. S. Drees, D. McDonald, J. Darracott,‡ E. J. Douglass,‡ B. H. R. Davenport, J. Donahue, J. Dean, M. Dillon, W. C. Daniel, P. D. Davis, H. Duparc, E. W. Davis, C. F. Daniels, H. W. Denslow, J. D. Delannoi, J. M. Dougherty, J. H. Dews, T. H. Dunham, R. Dinzey, E. J. Doyle, W. W. Doty, J. B. Davis, Samuel Douse, Chas. Davis,* W. J. Doggett, J. E. Demrard,‡ J. M. Doty, Daniel McDonald, Abner Doba, William Dougherty, John Dooner, Frank Doyle, Timothy Dorney, James Dolan, Barnard Dolan, Patrick Dignon, John J. Derrick, J. B. Davis,‡ Thomas D. Downing, Daniel Donahoe, Robert K. Dimond,† Philip J. DeLorge, Jas. Deasy, T. F. Daniel, R. A. Diehl, Richard Dawson,* John Dawson, M. Drury, J. J. Daly, P. F. Dillon, J. Duignan, Patrick Davis, P. Doyle, W. B. Devine, Thomas Daily, Ed. Dinnon,† Michael Dougherty, Daniel Doyle, John Duggan, M. Dohrman, C. Dreyer, Jacob G. Davis, H. DeDuring, Thomas H. Dunham,‡ George W. Dillon,† Raymond M. Demere, M. J. Donnelly, Patrick Dunn, Peter Derst,‡ John Derst, George Dieter, C. Drager, John Dunn,* John Dadwilder,† William Daunenfelser W. Dominey,‡ James Daniels,† E. B. Darden, J. T. Daniels, J. Danforth, M. Danforth, J. B. Davis,‡ R. A. Davis,‡ Henry Dugger,‡ John Denmark, Newton Davis, Jasper Davis,‡ John J. Davis†, P. Daley, J. Dillon, C. Dalton, J. C. Duke,† H. Demere, J. F. Davis, W. W. Dixon, W. H. Dean.

John Easter, Lewis Endres, H. A. Elkins, Lewis L. Eastmead,‡ J. H. Estill,‡ R. H. Elliott,† Percival Elliott,† S. Elliott, Jr., J. Eghlen, R. Exum, J. M. Elliott, J. W. Elliott, M. English, Maurice Erwin, Jefferson Espotons, William Elliott, J. S. Eden,† William Entwistle, A. Edmonds, J. L. Edmondson, A. Ehrlich,‡ George Ergil, F. Englehart, Nicholas Englehard, G. Erkil, W. R. Evans, Joseph Elarbee, M. Ennis, H. Eady,* William Eppinger, J. B. Ellis,* J. J. Eady, T. P. Elkins, J. W. Edmondson,* S. English.

John H. Forehand,‡ James L. Foster, Noah Folsom, M. E. Flowers, L. T. Flowers,† A. J. Franklin, M. H. Franklin,‡ Julius A. Ferrill,* Joseph M. Farr, T. C. Farr, L. A. Falligant, R. C. Feagan,† G. C. Freeman, J. T. Freeborn, E. N. Formsby, J. R. Farr, J. H. Frazier,† A. Fairchild, S. C. Freeman, W. H. Farrell, W. H. Ferguson, J. Fender, A. Folker,‡ M. L. Farris, W. B. Francis, R. R. Forbes,† J. C. Footman, J. A. Feuger, C. J. Falligant, John Fernandez, J. G. Fulton,† D. P. Freeman, F. S. Ferrill, James Freeborn, F. J. Fox, Patrick Flannery, John Foster, G. C. Fahm, M. F. Foley, Geo. G. Fathers,† Robert C. Felzer, R. Fetzer,‡ Wm. Foley, Robt. C. Fetzer, David Farmer, P. H. Ferguson, Thos. Feely, John Frain, R. Folliard,† Daniel Foley, Michael Fleming,‡ James Fleming, William Fowler, J. Fitzpatrick, James Farrell, Thomas H. Farrell, L. Freudenthal, Thos. Ferrill, L. Feuslenberg, J. S. Fisher, Dougald Ferguson, Joseph C. Faver, T. S. Flood, Wm. Frew,* John H. Fulton,† Fred. Ferrier, Jas. Ferguison,‡ F. Fisher,† E. B. Forbes, M. Floyd, R. J. Frizell, J. C. Fletcher, B. B. Farmer,† R. A. Fleming, A. Fitzpatrick, B. F. Fox, J. D. Ferguson, Robert C. Ferrill,‡ Lemuel A. Fryer, Richard Flinn, U. C. Frazier,* P. Fogarty, Wm. Fowler, I. Follard, I. Finn,† B. C. Ferguson,* J. D. Frazier, W. B. Fisher, W. J. Forehand, F. W. Finch, A. J. Franklin, W. H. Farmer, W. C. Flemister, J. M. Farr.

C. Gassman, J. Giddins, L. L. Graybill,‡ I. N. Grimes,‡ I. I. Griffin,‡ F. G. Goodwin,* R. J. Godfrey,‡ C. W. Godfrey, C. G. Girardeau,† F. A. Garden, J. B. Gaudry, A. T. Gray, C. Garrett, J. Gammell, Chas. A. Greiner,† John Golden, W.

G. Gray, E. J. Gowdy, N. E. Griffin, A. Goodman, W. J. Grubbs, H. F. Gilliland, John Gross, A. Goodman, S. P. Goodwin, E. L. Graves, B. J. Givoncelly, E. J. Gowdy, J. S. Gans,‡ E. Gordon, E. L. Gordon,† E. Griffin, B. Green,† R. D. Guerard, C. F. Grant, J. N. Guerard,† J. S. Griggs (drowned), H. Gallagher, C. W. Gould,† W. E. Guerard, S. D. Griffin, D. M. Gugel, H. L. Gilliland, W. S. Gowan, D. F. Goens, Thos. A. Grace, John Gribbin, Joseph Gammon, James Glenn, Geo. Grimshaw, Fleming Goldsby, John McGrath, Sr., John McGrath, Jr., August Gerber, M. Garritz, John J. Gallagher, Patrick Gahan, Patrick Gleason, James Golden, G. Geiger, William Gleeman, F. Green, G. Giebelhouse, G. Garey, B. L. Goulding, B. A. Grubbs, J. W. Graves, J. C. Gray, William Guisinheimer, Fisher Gaskins, James L. Griffin, Benjamin Green,† Robert C. Guerard,† Ed. Gordon, A. W. Graham,† F. R. Goulding, W. J. Grubbs, Frank Godwin, R. Garrison, W. Grimm, Wm. Gardner, John Geigher, S. Green,‡ John Gaskins, W. B. Gill, Thos. Gibbons, J. H. Geffcken, H. A. Gilbert, James Ginney,† J. V. Gray, J. N. Gow,† G. T. Gray, B. Gray, John T. Glatigny, Joshua Gnann, M. M. Glisson, James Gill, Wm. Gill, Silas H. Graves, R. Grant, T. H. Gibson, Wm. Groover, E. W. Gifford, A. W. Gresham, P. Guerard, A. G. Guerard, J. F. Gowen.

David Hutchinson,† Robert H. Hutchinson,‡ Alexander F. Holmes,‡ Jesse C. Heidt, E. L. Hacket, J. W. Heidt, R. R. Habersham, A. Holt, James Heery, G. T. Hetterick, A. T. Habersham,† John L. Harden, M. Haggerty, F. E. Hertz, H. P. Horton,† T. R. Hines, A. W. Harmon, Wm. Hays, W. H. Hudson, E. F. Henderson, M. Hamilton, C. M. Holst, B. M. Hunter, John Hughes, J. E. Henderson, J. B. Hogg, H. N. Heidt, W. Higgins, S. D. Hamilton, C. Hopkins, W. L. Haupt, F. J. Hunt,† T. Holcombe, F. W. Harriss, J. B. Harriss, J. Hitchcock, W. P. Hunter, S. O. T. Harvey, J. B. Holst, J. C. Holcombe, S. H. Hopkins,† T. Henderson, J. Harig, Thomas L. Henry, James H. Hull, N. A. Hardee,† J. F. Hamilton, W. R. Holmes, C. S. Harris, G. G. Hendrick, W. B. Hassett, E. R. Hernandez, B. J. Helny, Thomas Hinely,‡ W. N. Habersham,‡ W. C. Henges,‡ W. T. Ham, Albert Hunt, John Hodge, A. S. Hutchinson, E. B. Hook, W. Hutchinson,‡ John Hays, Henry Hastedtt, Wm. R. Hutchinson, Charles W. Harper, Henry Hinkins,† James Hourine,* Richard Hunt, W. O. Harper, John Hammond, Isaac Hay, Wm. Hernandez, F. A. Holliday, John Healey, Elijah J. Hall, George W. Hall, John Henry,* Patrick Hays, Stephen Hanlon,† Thos. Haley, J. Harrington, Bernard Horan, Patrick Hayes, Thos. Hymes,† C. Hartman, C. M. Harden, B. W. Hodgins, B. Hess, J. Hennings, D. Harmes, H. Harper, Charles Hennings, H. Hartloge, I. Harmes, H. Hartloe, John F. Hunter, George W. Hendrick, John Hart, J. W. Hendley, Samuel P. Hamilton, R. L. Hearn, T. W. Heyward,† Wm. H. Hewlitt, C. C. Hines, Jefferson Hyatt,‡ Thos. G. Heidt,* John Hess, Frank Hirt, C. Hirt, Wm. Haarer,‡ Henry Heine, Peter Hildebrandt, Wm. Haskel, S. Hernstadt,† B. Ham, D. Heusler, C. Heuer, Robt. Hurst,‡, John Howard,† Fred. Heuer,* H. Hicks, J. D. Howard,‡ James Halpine, L. Heuriant,† John Hinely,* Chas. Herb, R. M. Harris, James Hamlin, C. F. Hughes, J. Hanley, H. C. Harden,‡ W. J. Harris, W. J. Hulm, C. Hartman, J. E. Howard,* J. M. Harris, M. L. Harris, B. Horn, W. B. Heath, J. Hagerty,† J. M. Hills, Peter Hogan, James Higgins,‡ Jas. Hancock, W. S. Hancock, Alfred P. Horton, J. T. Hairgrooves, John Harris,† Jas. Hineley, S. Haughton,† A. Heery, M. Henry, C. H. Hamm, Alexander Hazzard,† Wm. Harden, R. P. Hoyt, T. R. Holliday, H. Humphreys, W. B. Hedleston, C. J. Hallman, H. M. Heidt, T. C. Harden, R. F. Harrington, J. R. Holtzclaw,* G. Harper, P. F. Hayden, G. H. Henning, J. B. Harrell.

Robt. Ivey, W. H. Ivey,† S. T. Isler,‡ Henry Inmen, John Inmen, C. F. Irwin, L. Ingalls, I. Ivey.

J. S. Jordan,† S. Jones,† E. C. Johnson, G. O. Johnson, W. Johnson, J. E. Jones, M. Joiner, J.W. Jaudon, J. Joiner, W. J. Jones, J. A. Johnston, F. P. Jones, A.Johnson, Mitchell Jones, T. Jones, H. B. Josephs, G. E. James,* P. Jordan,† R. Johnson, T. W. Johnson, B. L. Jones, J. B. Jones, J. Johnson (drowned), W. L. Jackson,‡ J. E. Jarrell, J. M. Jones, Jacob A. Jones, W. W. Jennings, Thomas Jennings, H. Jones, J. Jennings, F. Jackson, I. Johnson, P. E. Judine,† Samuel Jeffcoat,* Mathew Jones, Daniel J. Jones, H. H. Jones, Alfred Jones, Wm. A. Jaudon,* Wm. H. Jackson,‡ J. T. Jones, W. Jones, H. T. Johnson, T. G. Jones, J. H. Jones,‡ B. F. Jenkins, J. J. Johnson, O. Shelton Jinks,† J. H. Jackson,‡ M. Jackson, Wm. Johnson, W. B. Jackson, T. M. Jenkins, G. W. Johnson, C. Jolly.

P. Kreiger,‡ J. F. Krenson,* J. H. King,‡ M. Kelly, T. Kenny, M. L. King, A. D. Krenson, R. M. C. Kennedy, R. B. King, W. A. Keller,† E. H. Kent, R. King, E. J. Kirkland, T. King, F. Kreeger,‡ J. F. Kollock, G. J. Kollock, J. F. Kreeger,‡ J. M. Kreeger, N. B. Knapp, B. F. Keller, P. J. Kirby, J. Kirkland, J. A. M. King, L. Kelly, T. Kirby, R. H. Kennedy, D. S. Kellam, J. T. Knight, P. Kenane, T. Kearney, J. Kennedy,† J. Kinchen, J. A. King, Thos. Kelly, A. Kating, J. Kerns, J. Kavanagh, T. Kirby, Fred. Koch, H. Koch, F. Koch, P. Kelley, F. Krail, P. Koofman, J. Kuhlman, H. Kuck, F. M. Kinsey, B. Kennedy, A. Champion Knapp, S. Kraft,† Jacob Klein, George Knerr,† Wylly Knight,‡ John Kessell, Wm. Krauss, M. Kilner, C. Keller,† N. Kittrell, Wm. Kellum, James Keyes,‡ P. Kelley, E. J. Kennedy, T. Kile.

D. P. Landershine,† W. J. Lineberger, F. M. Lineberger,† W. N. Lineberger,† B. F. Lineberger,† B. F. Lindsey, J. R. M. Lindsey, J. S. Lindsey, Hardy Lovett,† Joshua Lovett, T. J. Liles,† J. R. Lewis, L. W. Landershine, Lewis Lippman,‡ J. Richard Lewis,* Samuel S. Law (murdered by negroes, on the Ogeechee road, the 3d of November, 1868, while gallantly resisting their advance upon the city), J. S. F. Lancaster, E. S. Lathrop, W. H. Lammon, W. W. Lincoln, William Lattimore, H. H. Linnville, J. W. Lathrop, T. H. Lyon, O. R. Lewis, L. J. Leconte, T. R. Lovell, W. H. Lamon, M. C. Lampe,† L. J. Lee, John Lee,* L. J. La Faucheur, G. W. Lavender, W. B. Lawton, D. F. Lafils, E. L. Lathrop, B. Ledley,† A. M. Lopez,* John Lamb, L. D. Lathrop, T. D. Lany,† G. Leonardy, John N. Lewis, C. A. Long,* O. A. Lavender,† H. M. Lufburrow, O. F. Lufburrow, Robt. Lachlison, Jr., Thos. Lyster, T. H. Laird, John Lynch, P. G. Lain, J. E. Lanier, Jesse Lee, T. H. Lane, Thos. McLane, [this soldier, during his imprisonment in Forts Delaware and Columbus, carried around his waist the silk banner presented to his company, Montgomery Guards, by the Sisters of Charity, and brought it safely to Savannah when exchanged. He died since the war], Joseph Leonardy, John Laffey, John D. Leigh,‡ J. Lorch, James Larkin, M. Lannon,† Jeremiah Leary, John Lovitt, Peter Lacy, P. Lenzer, J. Lohson, John T. Lathrop, I. Lenzer, John Leyton,† A. J. Lebey,† J. L. Legett, R. F. Lester, T. H. Lake, J. W. Langley (drowned while attempting to escape from Fort Powhatan), Wm. P. Lake, Daniel J. Lehy, J. Leggett,‡ James Leonard,‡ Henry Lindner,‡ C. Larcen,‡ Abraham Lane, E. R. Law, John Lynch, James L. Leonard, John Lightburn, Charles Lanning, James Lynch, J. H. Lee, G. F.Lambach, L. L. Lanier, James F. Lee, A. V. LaRoche, Berry Lane,* M. Lacy, J. M. B. Lesueur, H. C. Lanier,* J. J. Logan, W. W. Lanier, G. C. Lewis, A. B. LaRoche.

L. A. McCarthy, W. Matthis, J. M. Matthis, M. O. Messick, Wm. Matthis,‡ S.

D. Mabry, John Morrison, John Murphy, T. A. Murphy,‡ N. J. Money, George McSneed,† John M. Murray, L. J. McIntosh, P. Muller, W. J. Marshall, C. H. Morell, T. D. Morell, J. J. Meldrin, W. H. McDowell, L. J. Miller, W. H. McLeod, J. Maddox (drowned), J. E. Maxwell, W. P. Muller, M. McLaughlin,† C. R. Maxwell,‡ J. D. Munnerlyne, J. H. McIntosh,* A. P. Malloy,* J. P. McIntyre, J. McCann, S. Millette, S. H. Manning, G. R. McRae, E. W. Miller, J. S. McDonnell, A. W. Mannell, C. M. Miller, D. McDonald, V. Martin, R. W. Miller, J. McGrath, A. McAlpine, J. C. Munnerlyne, W. H. C. Mills, Richard Millen,* J. W. Myddelton,* John Maker,* J. C. McNulty, Oscar McClusky,† P. H. Minis, S. L. Morton,* E. McComack, S. E. Myddelton, A. McAlpine, R. Mutall, M. Mahon, A. C. Miller, T. P. Miller, R. D. Millen, B. L. McIntosh,‡ M. McLean,‡ Geo. F. Mell, A. McHale, L. E. McCarthy, P. J. Mullarky, T. A. Miller, Daniel Moses, Jas. Maxwell, John McCormick,† A. P. Moon, W. F. May, Charles Moore, J. H. Morris,† John Mason, D. Mason, Allen Moody,† H. McMillen, Chas. Mortimer, H. C. Miller, Joseph Mansfield, D. C. Murphy, J. F. McGrath, N. Moore, A. Martin, J. Meaghin, T. Mulligan, W. H. McLeary, J. T. McDuff,* A. McDermott, F. McFeeley, J. N. Moore, A. Meyer, W. Manning, J. Morrison,† J. Masterson, H. Martin, H. Miller, J. R. Minnis, T. H. McGrath, B. McCarthy,† T. McElline, Francis McCann, T. McGinnis, J. H. McCann, T. McCann, J. McColloch, R. McKeone, J. McDonald, Ed. McNichols,* Jas. McGowan,‡ Andrew McGriel,‡ Timothy Murray.

T. D. Neely,† W. P. Newman, B. Newbern,† B. M. Neely, W. R. Norris, T. Neasing, T. N. Newall, T. J. Naylor, J. Nicholson, Patrick Noon,† Thomas C. Nieny, Frederick Nohr, T. S. Norton, J. H. Nesmith,† E. L. Nease, Thomas Newton, Henry Nelson, W. T. Nash, John Nicholson, J. R. Norton, S. Newman.

G. W. Osmond, J. Osmond, jr.,‡ W. H. Overstreet,† T. O'Neal, H. H. O'Farrell, T. A. Owens, Jas. O'Brien, T. O'Leary, P. O'Leary, M. O'Callahan, Dennis O'Quigley, James O'Connell, Michael O'Connor, Patrick O'Reily, Daniel O'Sullivan, Thos. O'Hara, O. Owens, Robt. Ornsby, George Outten,† J. H. O'Byrne, M. C. O'Grady, John Obsen, H. D. Ogletree, John W. Osteen, Wm. S. Owen, M. J. O'Brien, Jas. L. O'Byrne, Patrick O'Brien,‡ M. O'Byrne, Patrick O'Brien.

H. M. Parnell,‡ Thomas Purse, Jr.,* B. S. Purse, W. M. Patterson,* P. Prenty, T. G. Pond, J. J. Prendergast,* Clavius Phillips, J. A. Page, Francis Patat, J. E. Page, W. C. Patten, S. J. Perry,† James Partington, Charles B. Patterson, E. A. Parker, E. A. Pappy,† C. B. Postell,† P. Pardue,† E. P. Postell,* W. Pope, T. Purse, W. Pearson, Edward Paine, A. E. Patterson, P. D. Phelan,* Ira Payne, J. Peal, J. Pyne, C. J. Pratt, John H. Pacetti, M. B. Pindar, B. J. Pacetti, John T. Pacetti, J. F. Padrick, J. H. Polk,‡ T. P. Peck, C. J. Pratt, J. C. Prendergast, J. M. B. Pajay, M. Peyton, M. G. Prendergast, R. A. Pacetti, Dennis Pacetti, George Sweat, C. A. Patello, F. G. Pacetti, J. H. Polk, N. T. Pinder, J. B. Pinder, T. P. Peck, James Postell, R. A. Pollard, James G. Pournelle, J. A. Parrish,† E. A. Parrish, H. T. Parrish,† H. J. Parrish, Sion H. Pike,† Jno. Paulk,* John Pierce,† Thomas Peel, W. C. Patten, A. Ponce,† J. H. Peck.

G. T. Quantock, J. C. Quinn, P. Quinan, H. Quinne,* J. Quinan, H. J. Quantock,† Jasper N. Rogers, Wm. H. Rose,‡ Bradford Ray,‡ James L. Rowntree,† Hiram Ray,* J. Robinson, C. J. Ridding, J. C. Reynolds, R. W. Rawlston, W. H. Rice,* R. S. Register, J. T. Ray, G. B. Rice, B. J. Rouse,* M. Rowe,† J. B. Roberts, E. F. T. Roland, John Rielly, J. A. Reynolds, F. Rayes, A. M. Richards, J. B. Ripley, G. Robertson, R. R. Richards, J. Rains, J. T. Roland, J. Rosse, E. A. Rohrer, W. R. Roberts, Geo. Rose, Alex. Raymur, George R. Robertson, J. P. Rockley, John Roberts, J. M. Roberts, G. C. Roberts, John G. Rice, Aaron Rice,

J. A. Raulerson, E. T. Rogers, F. Rogers, Ed. Rielly,† Francis Roache, M. Redmond, H. Roberts, M. Reily, Jno. Reily, W. R. Ross, O. Roche,† Jas. Reed,† Jno. Robinson, Danl. Reily, Jas. Reily, F. Reily, James Redmond, J. F. Rotzer, H. W. Rockner, A. L. Robider,‡ C. R. Read, Noah Roe, W. J. Rickerson, Z. B. Reid, Oscar W. Reid, L. L. Richardson, L. R. Robey, J. W. Rahn,* Daniel Rambo, Thos. Robinson, Mitchell Roberts,† Elisha Roberts,† Hiram Richardson, David Roos, J. Red, I. Rahn,* M. Ryan, P. Rourke,† J. Robothams,† H. A. Rawlings, W. B. Riley, W. G. Rye, J. Rothwell,† C. D. Rogers, T. C. Reyes, I. Rice, M. Rodgers, S. P. Rape,† S. W. Ryan, R. W. Rice, M. W. Rice, J. C. Robbins, J. M. Roberts, J. T. Rahn, C. W. Rogers, W. H. Roberts, E. S. Remington, J. Richardson, jr., J. H. Rossignoll, C. H. Reid, W. C. Remshart, C. Roberts,† J. Rafferty,† M. Redmond.†

W. C. Shed (drowned), Gilbert H. Sneed, Wm. N. Sneed, James Sullivan, John Shellman, A. L. Shellman, A. H. Shaw,‡ Ashley M. Shaw,‡ Charlton H. Shaw, Peter U. Sineath, Geo. W. Sineath, Joseph J. Singuer,* Fred. Sheahan,† W. D. Sullivan, H. F. Symons, W. F. Symons,‡ H. Scrott, L. Salvatere, Eugene Stiles, S. S. Sessions, J. Santrefit, P. H. Santrefit, J. T. Stone, F. R. Sweat,‡ C. J. Sweat, Geo. Sweat, F. Stanwood, J. A. Santina,* S. Sturtevant, John Sullivan, John Sheridan,† W. S. Smith,† John Smith,‡ J. Taylor Smith,‡ S. Syntis,‡ D. R. Stevens,† H. Snyder, W. W. Smith, L. H. Shephard, W. E. Skinner, C. Steuart, P. B. Shay, B. Stonin, J. T. Stone, C. Schlatter, G. P. Screven, D. W. C. Spencer, C. A. Stiles, W. Starr, S. V. Stiles, J. Shaw, W. C. Stayley, G. R. Smith, W. L. Shaffer, W. G. Solomon, A. L. Sammons,‡ J. S. Spear, J. Sammons,† A. Sapp,† T. Smith,† J. F. Slade, C. Subcraft, L. Sheridan, M. Shea, B. Sneed, F. H. Spence, A. M. Smith, J. Stroud,† G. Simpson, G. W. Strous,† G. F. Seagers, I. Seagers,‡ F. F. Sapp, Lawrence Sullivan, John A. Stevenson, James Saunders, J. Stevenson,† B. Stevenson, E. Scudder, John Schroeder, Thomas Stone,† J. Simpson, B. Starke, J. Shine, R. Simms, Cornelius Sullivan, John Sullivan, J. T. Smith, D. Sullivan, O. Sullivan, James Sullivan, D. P. Sullivan, Hugh Smith, M. Schine,† Mortimer Shea, Michael Scott, R. J. Smith, E. G. Saussy,† J. B. Sibley, C. A. Sagurs, S. Sumner, A. C. Sumner, A. Seaman,† A. J. Sammons, E. W. Sammons,† W. Sumner, W. A. Simpson,† John Simpson, G. N. Saussey,‡ John A. Sullivan, E. A. Silva,‡ J. V. Smith, George M. Salfner, M. O. Scott,* H. H. Sharp, C. Schmanch, W. Stephen, C. Shafer,‡ P. Shafer, J. Selzer,† L. Snee, H. Sheer, F. Schreider, H. Schmidt, J. Schmidt, J. Steppens, J. C. Stephens, W. Smith,‡ A. N. Smith, J. Spell, A. Stokes, T. V. Stokes, A. W. Stokes, J. Stokes, P. Stone, A. B. Stone, E. M. Stibbs, Wm. Skippen,‡ H. E. Snider, David Smith, N. H. Saxon, A. B. Saxon, T. B. Sullivant, M. Sullivan, — Speisseger, J. D. Strobhart, James Smith, W. H. Snider, G. W. Shackelford, I. Smith, W. Smith, C. L. Schreck, B. Sanders, E. J. Stone, L. J. Sturdivant,* John W. Smith,* Patrick Sullivan, Wm. Strother,† Benj. Stokes,† W. Shannon,† J. L. Springs,† W. Snedeker, B. F. Syms, G. Street,† R. W. Skipper,† W. F. Sewell,* T. Smith, C. S. Smith, M. Smith, J. J. Smith, A. C. Scott, jr., H. M. Stoddard, S. H. Stewart, R. B. Slater, J. J. Shephard, H. M. Stoddard, R. B. Sandiford,‡ B. J. Strickland,† J. A. Sweat, G. W. Stevens, F. A. Sturtevant,‡ W. B. Sturtevant,‡ George P. Snider, J. F. Stone, S. A. Shell, Julius J. Smith, Lewis A. Sessions, Jas. E. Sweat,‡ Henry Stibbs, Wesley Smith, J. R. Saussy, M. Slammon, C. Smith, J. H. Silva, F. R. Stone, W. G. Spence, J. L. Solomons, R. W. Stubbs, Lewis Smith, Wm. Sumner, W. H. Sykes, J. S. Silva, A. W. Silva, J. M. Simpson, C. H. Saussy, H. Smith, jr., C. Smith, P. Siney.

George W. Tennant, Chas. H. Thiot,† L. T. Theus, W. A. Thomas, I. L. Toole, H. Truchelut, G. T. Theus, R. H. Tatem, Josiah Tattnall, H. J. Thomason, L. E.

Tebeau, W. Taylor, George Taylor,† L. Thomas, I. Tyree, S. L. Templeton, J. B. Thornton, P. Tippens, M. Thornton,† J. M. Thomas,† Patrick Tiernay, Patrick Tracey, Charles H. R. Thorpe, M. Tidwell, H. Tillman, John Triay, Francis B. Tarver, Wm. Thompson, Jno. Tobin, Francis R. Taylor, S. B. Terrill, P. Terry, P. Tigh, Pat. Tuberty, J. H. Tamm, J. Tyler, B. H. Theus,‡ B. Turner, Andrew Teynac, Jno. F. Teynac, J. M. Tuten,† H. Tuten,† W. Tuten,† Henry Turner,* Wm. C. Thomas,‡ S. B. Torlay,† Roland Terry, James Toole, F. E. Tebeau,† H. J. Templeton, J. H. Theatt, W. Taylor, J. Tant, J. J. Thompson, O. J. Tooles, S. T. Thompson,‡ J. H. Tooles, T. B. Tutle,* W. P. Trutt,* J. S. Turner,* E. J. Trutt, W. A. Templeton, G. J. Thomas, R. Tutle, J. R. Thompson, J. C. Thompson, R. B. Thompson,‡ A. R. Tinsley,‡ C. H. Thiot,† J. D. Tenbroeck, A. V. Toole, J. Tiernay, A. Tomlinson, H. B. Trist, T. N. Theus, W. C. Tuggle, L. W. Thompson, J. C. Toler, J. M. J. Thompson, George Turner.

M. C. Ulmer, G. C. Ulmer, J. D. Underwood,† G. C. Underwood,‡ Sanchez Usina, Charles Unus, J. T. Ulmer.

J. C. Veitch, John Volber, J. Vitchen, W. G. Vaughan, Henry VanGiesen, J. R. Valleau, William Van Horn, John H. Vincent, Jesse Vaughan, W. N. Valleau.†

James W. Williams, William D. Williams,† Griffin E. Williams, James M. Williams, E. Berney Williams, John F. White, James H. White,† John C. Wright, James R. Wells,† Lewis B. Wells,† D. R. Willis, J. C. Whittington,‡ Charles Weaver, J. T. Wells, J. J. Ward, J. Wilborne, A. Watson, F. N. Wilkinson, C. N. West, A. C. Walsh, W. Woodward, H. H. Woodbridge, R. W. Woodbridge, I. Washburne, U. P. Wade, O. D. Watson,† G. C. Wilson, E. C. Wade,† D. Wells, A. C. Wright, A. P. Wright, Frank Willis, George Waters,† J. T. Weldon,* C. L. Whitehurst, H. Waddell, T. C. Whitehurst, J. P. Williamson, A. M. Wood,* V. Walsh, J. Wylly,† J. M. Wylly,† George Woods, John Wallace, Martin Wall, Thomas Waters,† Edward Wright, James Williams, Lester Wallack, John Welsh, Charles Wood, Thomas Waters,† Alexander Williams, H. White, W. B. Wright, Thomas Walker, Charles White, William Woods, A. Waters,† P. Whitty, P. Walsh, James Willis, J.. J. Walsh,† William Walsh, Maurice Walsh, Edward Walsh, Dennis Walsh,‡ Jeremiah Walsh, Edward Wickham, C. Wigand, G. D. Wigand, Jno. Welsh, Jno. Wiggins,‡ K. C. Williams, W. D. Weaver, Berrien White, W. W. West, Frank White, E. G. Wilson,† James Wall,† W. W. Waddell, R. K. Walker, J. L. Way, A. R. Waller, R. Wilkerson, — Ward,† L. Werm,‡ M. Williams,‡ W. C. Williams, John Waston, S. Wilson, John Ward, L. Watts,† John Willis,† James Winslow, H. Wise, A. Watson, G. W. Williams,† John Welsh,* Thomas A. Wilson,* T. E. Waldron, C. Whittel, J. P. K. Walker, J. R. Wray,‡ T. J. White, George W. Williams,† James Welsh, P. Winbern, Hiram Waller,‡ Thaddeus Waller, William Waller, Thomas Watters,* T. Welch, E. Williams, G. C. Wood, A. Watson, P. White, A. Williams, H. W. Wise, I. Wood, J. W. Weed, W. B. Woodbridge, R. W. Wall, F. M. Wall, J. M. Waters, J. M. Weatherly,‡ J. S. Weatherly, H. J. Wade, B. C. Wagner,† E. H. Williams, T. S. Wilson, M. Wiggins, J. H. Watson, F. M. Willis, E. P. Wait, P. C. Wiggins, J. P. Webb, S. Walls, W. L. Wakelee, John Webb,† John H. Wright,‡ J. P. Williamson, William E. White, A. M. West, G. W. Wilkes,† G. P. Walker, C. W. West, Joseph Washburn, R. G. Williams, John Wilkes, F. M. Walker, J. N. Wasden, M. J. Williams, Solomon Wilkes, J. J. Wilkes, G. B. Willet, W. B. Wylly, William Wade, W. A. Walker.

Henry Younge, Frank Yeager, I. Young, D. Yates, William Yokum, William Young, J. P. Young,* A. J. Young, James Yokum.

D. Zittrouer, L. H. Zachary, E. S. Zittrouer, G. Zehubauer, G. A. Zittrouer.

SAVANNAH AS IT IS.

Stretching along the southern bank of the Savannah river stands Savannah, the Forest City of the South. A sandy plain, fifty feet above the level of the sea, and about eighteen miles by the course of the river from it, is its site. This plateau, upon which the city rests, is almost a level, being forty-eight feet above the level of the sea at the Pulaski House, fifty feet at the intersection of Montgomery and Gwinnett streets, and forty-six feet at the Park; at this point and level commences a ridge or back-bone of dry pine land, extending due south and aptly marked by the White Bluff road, which curiously divides the waters of the Ogeechee from the waters of the Vernon rivers. This ground was originally covered with dense forests, which were cleared away very soon after the introduction of the Royal government in 1752. The city is open and spacious, being divided by numerous and wide streets and lanes intersecting each other at right angles, with large squares at regular distances, adding much to the beauty and health of the city. In addition to the squares there is a large park (Forsyth Place), embracing ten acres of land, laid off in the southern part of the city. The city is well supplied with water and lighted with gas.

The Savannah river, soon after passing the city in its course to the ocean, is divided into numerous channels by small islands of marsh, the beautiful and delicate green of which, interspersed in the waters, affords, when viewed from the northeastern extremity of the bluff on a summer afternoon, one of the softest scenes imaginable.

There is an area of country, determined by two measurements—a north and south line of nine to ten miles in length and an east and west line of about the same length which must be of great future interest to the well-wishers and actual inhabitants of the city of Savannah. This area lies between the Savannah river as a northern limit, the Ogeechee and Vernon rivers, with their tributaries, as a southern limit, the St. Augustine creek and Vernon river as an eastern limit, and the great tide-water swamp stretching due south from the Savannah to the Ogeechee river as a western limit. The thorough and complete drainage of this Mesopotamia, now in contemplation, would add untold wealth to its people and render their sanitary condition the most enviable in the world.

This area, on the mid-northern edge of which Savannah rests, is bisected by an elevated piny ridge, upon which run the White Bluff and Middle Ground roads. All the waters of the eastern slopes of this water-shed empty into the Vernon river, through a swamp about seven miles long and extending from the Catholic cemetery, on the Thunderbolt road, to the tide-water of Vernon river at Hanner's bridge ; and all the waters of the western slopes of this water-shed empty into the Ogeechee river, through a great swamp extending from the dam or back-water of the Springfield plantation to this river's channel. Thus this area is drained by two long swamps, whose waters belong severally to the Vernon and Ogeechee rivers.

It is worthy of note that this western swamp, with all its multitudinous ramifications, is a tide-water swamp, subject to a greater or less influx and efflux of water at each tide, and stretching from the Savannah river to the Ogeechee. Between these points there is a gradual rise of the land to a *summit level* three to five feet above mean high-water mark, and about the three-mile stone of the Ogeechee plank roak, from which summit level the waters have a natural tendency to flow north to the Savannah river and south to the Ogeechee. This fact was demonstrated by the inundation of the Springfield plantation at the time of Sherman's advance upon the city. The swamp waters were backed up to a level five feet above high-water mark, and would have escaped into the Ogeechee swamp and river but for a dam three feet high erected by the engineer department in a short narrow swamp connecting the two great swamps. This is in striking contrast to the Vernon River swamp, which has a steady rise of fourteen feet to the Catholic cemetery. This extensive tide-water swamp is uncleared and uncultivated in its whole extent, except immediately upon the western edge of the city of Savannah, where before the year 1820 (the date of the dry-culture contract) an extremely valuable rice plantation existed, stretching from the river front to a back-water dam, built by the original owner, Joseph Stiles, an Oglethorpe colonist. This dam is parallel with the most extended southern limit of the city. Unhappily for Savannah the dry-culture contract caused an entire abandonment of these once cultivated swamp-lands, and in consequence the ditches, canals, dams, trunks, and gates have all gone to decay, and the last condition of them is ten-fold worse than the first. To increase the embarrassment, the high embankments of the Central railroad and Ogeechee canal divide this plantation in two parts, on the line of Liberty street, and thus permanently intercept the natural lines of drainage. This Springfield plantation contains five hundred acres, and is a narrow belt of low land three hundred yards wide.

These obstacles to the drainage of these lands are, however, formidable only because of the cost of culverting the canal and railroad embankments. The outlet of the water has a descent, at low water, of six feet, and is, therefore, easy and not involving a great expense. It is a pleasure and encouragement to the despondent in this matter to recall the draining of the Alban lake by Camillus in the early days of Rome A. U. 350, with its wonderful tunnel or Emissary through the living rock, two and a half miles long, to remember the draining of Lake Velinus into the Nar by Curius Dentatus, A. U. 460, who thus created the beautiful falls of Terni, one hundred and forty feet high, and thus drained thirty square miles of territory; and the draining of Lake Fucinus into the Liris by the Emperor Claudius by an Emissary three miles long, and part of it through carnelian rock. The outlet to the water of Springfield is six feet below the level of the land, and in contrast it is well to call to mind the draining of Harlem lake, thirty-three miles in circumference, covering forty-five thousand three hundred acres of land, with a water outlet to the sea twenty feet above the lake—a work begun in 1836 and completed in 1852.

Being a short distance from the sea, and no barrier intervening, the regular sea breezes easily penetrate to the city, and are received every day, unless an accidental counter-current of wind prevents it. They are delightful and refreshing at all times during the summer, and, in consequence of the thorough drainage of the last three years to the east and southeast of the city, can be considered at all times wholesome. These breezes are constant and almost unremitting during the day time in the months of August and September.

Savannah is in 32 degrees and some minutes of latitude, with the Gulf Stream just issuing from the tropics at no great distance to the eastward. It is near the isothermal line of 70 degrees mean temperature, which marks the northern limit of the tropics. The mean temperature of Savannah is 66 degrees, and nearly approaches the temperature of Bermuda, 68 degrees; Gibraltar, Spain, 64 degrees; Palermo, Sicily, 66 degrees; Shanghai, China, 66 degrees; Montevideo, S. A., 66 degrees; Cape Town, Africa, 65.8 degrees; Sydney, Australia, 64.6 degrees.

These circumstances, together with the radiating quality of the surface of the soil, rendered it in former times very hot. At the present day the heats of summer have fallen off to a remarkable degree. It is seldom that the temperature exceeds 85 degrees in May, 90 degrees in June, and 92 degrees in August and September. It is hardly necessary to remind the reader that the heated term of six weeks north and northwest of the Potomac and Ohio rivers exhibits a temperature from 95 degrees to 105 degrees. The summer comprehends more than one half of the year; it usually commencences in May, and may be said not to terminate until November. For although some cool weather occurs in September and October, it is slight and prevails chiefly during the nights. The cold of winter is not steadily established before the latter part of December or beginning of January. Before that time it fluctuates very much. It does not continue steadily beyond the month of February; and even in this month the peach tree and jessamine have put forth their blossoms; so that the duration of winter, strictly considering it, does not exceed six weeks.

The reproach of Savannah is a mild malarial poisoning of the atmosphere existing from April to November. But the intense malaria which formerly made July, August, and September a terror both to strangers and natives, and gave to these months the title "sickly months," has almost totally ceased. High grade bilious fevers are almost unknown, and congestive chills and congestive fevers have been extremely rare in the last three years. During this period the very slight mortality of the summer months has been truly remarkable. With a population of forty-five thousand the average number of deaths, whites and colored, was nineteen for each week of August, 1868, and thirty for each week of September, 1868. Measles and scarlet fever have been almost unknown in the past three years. Typhoid fevers were unrecognized in the category of diseases in Savannah before 1850. Since that time they have occasionally occurred. During the recent war this class of disease occurred very constantly in the experience of physicians. Immediately after the fall of Savannah, and for some months subsequently, very violent cases of cerebro-spinal meningetis occurred in the city.* At the present time it may be safely asserted that typhoid fevers are extremely rare. Puerperal fevers and puerperal accidents, so common in the northern cities, are comparatively unknown to our female population. Cholera infantum, that scourge of children in the Northern cities, is only known by its exceptional occurrence. Consumption does occasionally originate in Savannah, but always under the powerful depressing agency of (*not cold as in the North*) malaria. It is an accepted fact in the medical world that an equable temperature is as important to the unfortunate consumptive as warmth, and in this particular, from the middle of February to the first of December, Savannah recommends itself remarkably; for, during this period of nearly ten months of the year, the ranges of temperature are from 70 degrees to 92 degrees, and this variation of 22 degrees is at all times very easy and gradual. Until the Springfield plantation is drained, however, the prevalence of a mild malarial depression must render Savannah undesirable for the consumptive.

As each succeeding summer opens upon the city, a vague apprehension seizes the minds of her people that an epidemic of yellow fever may be ushered in. Such an apprehension is a misfortune in itself: it argues the belief that this disease has been the constant concomitant of past summers. This belief is erroneous, as a simple and brief record may readily show. Up to 1820 there is no record of the disease. That it may have existed sporadically and unrecognized before this date can not be denied. There is extant a letter of Dr. William R. Waring, a well-known physician of Savannah, of date 1819, to the distinguished investigator of yellow fever, Dr. Churvin, in which he expresses the belief that yellow fever is only a high grade bilious fever. Needless to add that this opinion was changed in the very next year, when occurred the epidemic of 1820. It commenced on the 5th of September and was checked on the 6th of November. The number of deaths were two hundred

* After the fall of Savannah Sherman's army, numbering about seventy-five thousand men and an enormous number of animals, remained for a month or two within or near the city limits. During the months of February and March the scavenger department, organized by the United States authorities, moved from the interior of the city proper five hundred and sixty-eight dead animals, eight thousand three hundred and eleven cart loads of garbage, and seven thousand two hundred and nineteen loads of manure. To these accumulations of deleterious material may be attributed the sickness of that period.

and thirty-nine. Not a case is recorded until the epidemic of 1827, which was comparatively trifling. From 1830 to 1839 not a case occurred in the city. In this year an epidemic occurred in Augusta and Charleston, and a few cases were brought to Savannah. The year 1839 was one of the sickliest ever known in Savannah. It is remembered as the dryest summer on record, and also a very hot summer. Bilious fevers prevailed in a malignant form, but not yellow fever. In 1840 and 1841 sporadic cases are recorded, but from 1843 to 1852 no more cases. In 1852 and 1853 sporadic cases were noted, and then followed the epidemic of 1854, which commenced on the 3d of August and was checked during the first week of November. The number of deaths were 1040.

August, whites........... 235; blacks........................ 22
September, whites....... 591; blacks........................ 55
October, whites......... 108; blacks........................ 29

Of the above the following were from yellow fever:

August, whites........... 132; blacks........................ 1
September, whites....... 381; blacks........................ 9
October, whites......... 67; blacks........................ 4

It is computed that these deaths occurred in a population of six thousand who remained to brave the epdemic.*

In each succeeding year after this date rare sporadic cases occurred until there broke out the epidemic of 1858, which, in comparison with that of 1854, was trifling, there being only one hundred and fifteen deaths from this cause. There were a few cases in 1861, since which date three, or at most four, sporadic cases have been mentioned in medical circles.

In brief, since the publication of the able work of LeRoche, the universal belief of the medical fraternity is, that the *cause* of yellow fever is of local origin, and produced by a poison—the mixed result of the exhalations or emanations of decaying vegetable and animal matters, which separately produce the well-known varieties of malarial and typhoid diseases.

---

* A very large number of the deaths are set down as having occurred from other diseases than yellow fever. A great number of cases of yellow fever resulted fatally, the immediate cause being the development of constitutional and other complications of disease. The physicians, in making their reports, gave the immediate cause of the deaths, without mentioning the attack of fever by which the patient had been prostrated. The systems of persons who have had the fever are very much exposed to the fatal ravages of other diseases during the tedious and precarious process of recovery.

It may now safely be predicted that the great expansion of the city proper, thorough scavenger's work and thorough drainage will in the future prevent yellow fever in Savannah as thoroughly as it has in Philadelphia.

THE COMMERCIAL INTERESTS AND ADVANTAGES OF SAVANNAH.

The harbor of Savannah is capacious and well protected. The bar, outside of the mouth of the river, is about twenty miles from the city, and has on it a greater depth of water than on any on the Southern coast.* The channel is from a half to three quarters of a mile in width. Just inside of the bar is situated Tybee island, abreast of which, about four miles from the bar, is good anchorage in five to six fathoms of water. From this anchorage-ground to Venus Point (nine miles from the city) there is a depth of nineteen feet, and from the Point to the city seventeen feet of water.

There is a floating light off "Martin's Industry," about fifteen miles northeast of Tybee, moored in six fathoms; two light-houses on Tybee island, the principal one of which is on a structure one hundred and fifty-two feet high, the other is a beacon light fifty-six feet high; a light-house on Cockspur island, five miles inside of the bar, and another on the oyster-beds, six miles inside; and another on the eastern end of Fig island. There are also lights placed at the obstructions in the river, and another upon the eastern end of the bluff.

The limited amount of wharf front to the city will in a short time necessitate an increased accommodation to meet the wants of the growing commerce of the city. General Edward C. Anderson, the Mayor of the city, in his annual report, refers to this want, and says that sufficient accommodation can be attained by an extension of the line of wharves below Willink's ship-yard, where the water is deep, or, by means of the powerful dredge machine now in the river, widening, deepening, and wharfing the Ogeechee canal from the lock to the Central Railroad bridge, and converting it into a basin for ships. The distance between the two points named is three thousand and seventy-eight feet on either bank, amounting to six thousand one hundred and fifty-six feet in all, or an equivalent

* About thirty years ago a committee was appointed by the Secretary of the Navy to examine the bars from Charleston, S. C., to St. Marys, Ga., and reported: "The bar at the mouth of the Savannah river is the deepest and most accessible of any on the Southern coast. The average depth is nineteen feet at low water; hence with a full tide (twenty-five feet) a frigate may pass in safety."

of nearly one mile and a quarter of additional wharf accommodation to the city. The present width of the canal is one hundred and thirty feet, which, without difficulty, could be increased to one hundred and eighty feet, or two hundred feet, and deepened to any extent that might be deemed desirable. The project is suggested for the consideration of capitalists. Judiciously carried out, and with a line of rail track on either side of the basin running up to the railroad bridge from the river, it would afford an admirable location for the Cotton Presses, and doubtless prove a profitable investment to all parties undertaking it, as well as an essential accommodation to the prospective business interests of Savannah.

Shortly after the settlement of Savannah she became of considerable importance along the Atlantic coast, and previous to the Revolutionary war her exports became somewhat equal to her natural advantages. Not, however, until the advent of cotton culture was her position assumed, and for many years after its introduction her older rival, Charleston, overshadowed her efforts at advancement, controlling, by her enterprise and wealth, a larger portion of the sea island, and the whole of the Florida trade, and even penetrating through the inland route to the rice lands around Savannah, the products of which were in many instances sent there for sale. Up to the building of the Central railroad, Savannah was behind her more wealthy neighbor, and even long after, but it soon became apparent that the new road was to give Savannah an impetus not to be rivalled if properly fostered. Thus year by year, as road after road was completed, opening up the State and pouring its products into the lap of Savannah, her merchants reaped the reward due them for their foresight, zeal, and enterprise, which have made their city the second cotton port of the country.

The permanent establishment of the line of steamers from Savannah to Liverpool will materially assist in developing this city and Georgia, and every encouragement should be given to the enterprise by the merchants and business men in all parts of Georgia, and by our railroads. Another project for which the capitalists of Savannah must bid, is the Southern Pacific railroad, of which some survey is now being made. The northern route is found to be beset with difficulties in winter, and the parties interested in the road are looking toward the establishing of the southern line with a great degree of interest. Their attention, and that of others interested, is called to the article on the subject under the head of "The Central Railroad."

DEVELOPMENT OF RESOURCES.

The course of Savannah is manifestly onward, and with the exercise of that energy the proud monuments of which are seen on every hand, will shortly place her in the position to which she is entitled by her fine harbor, her railroads, and the extensive and fertile back country, the products of which must find exit from her harbor.

The gradual development of the resources of Savannah will be exhibited by the following figures, showing her exports for the years 1749, 1750, 1753, 1763, 1773, 1786, 1796, 1800, 1818, 1821, 1825 1826, 1839, 1840, 1841, 1842, 1843, 1844, 1845, 1846, 1847, 1854, 1855, 1856, 1857, 1858, 1859, 1860, 1865, 1866, 1867, 1868:

In 1749, when the first exports from the colony were made, the value was $10,000.

In 1750, the exports amounted in value to $8,897.

In 1753, 2,996 barrels of rice, 9,395 pounds of indigo, 268 pounds of silk, which, with the peltry, lumber, and provisions exported, amounted in value to $74,785.

In 1763, 7,500 barrels of rice, 9,633 pounds of indigo, 5,000 bushels of indian corn, a large quantity of lumber, peltry, and provisions were exported, amounting in value to $193,395.

In 1773, the value of exports was $379,422.

In 1786, the value was $321,377.

In 1796, $501,383.

In 1800, $2,155,982.

In 1818,* $14,183,113.

In 1821, $6,032,862.

The following statement shows the amount of the staple articles exported to foreign ports and coastwise:

In 1825, 64,906 bags of cotton, and 2,154 tierces of rice, foreign; 72,789 bags of cotton, and 5,081 tierces of rice, coastwise.

In 1826, 108,486 bags of cotton, and 4,978 tierces of rice, foreign; 82,092 bags of cotton, and 6,477 tierces of rice, coastwise.

In 1839, 199,176 bags of cotton, and 21,322 tierces of rice.

In 1840, 284,249 bags of cotton, and 24,392 tierces of rice.

---

* In 1818 the exports were larger and the articles commanded a higher price than at any previous time, and for many years afterward. The large decrease in the number, and consequently the value of the exports in 1821, is due to the yellow fever in the fall of 1820, during which all business was suspended, and from the effects of which the business interests of the city did not recover for a year or two. The imports in 1818 were valued at $2,976,257, and in 1821 at $865,146.

In 1841, 147,280 bags of cotton, 23,587 tierces of rice, and 14,295,-200 feet lumber.

In 1842, 142,386 bags of cotton, 5,933 tierces of rice, and 5,919,-400 feet of lumber, foreign; 79,868 bags of cotton, 16,131 tierces of rice, and 2,471,000 feet of lumber, coastwise.

In 1843, 193,099 bags of cotton, 10,675 tierces of rice, and 5,532,-750 feet of lumber, foreign; 87,727 bags of cotton, 15,606 tierces of rice, and 1,986,800 feet of lumber, coastwise.

In 1844, 130,964 bags of cotton, 10,307 tierces of rice, and 3,034,-064 feet of lumber, foreign; 113,611 bags of cotton, 18,236 tierces of rice, and 2,889,187 feet of lumber, coastwise.

In 1845, 182,073 bags of cotton, 11,712 tierces of rice, and 3,333,-646 feet of lumber, foreign; 122,471 bags of cotton, 17,505 tierces of rice, and 4,936,936 feet of lumber, coastwise.

In 1846, 77,852 bags of cotton, 5,025 tierces of rice, and 13,365,-968 feet of lumber, foreign; 108,454 bags of cotton, 27,122 tierces of rice, and 5,219,676 feet of lumber, coastwise.

In 1847, 119,321 bags of cotton, 10,218 tierces of rice, and 48,-886,425 feet of lumber, foreign; 114,830 bags of cotton, 21,521 tierces of rice, and 5,844,960 feet of lumber, coastwise.

In 1854, 98,580 bales of upland, and 3,861 bales of sea island cotton, foreign; 203,363 bales of upland, and 11,667 bales of sea island cotton, coastwise—total value, $15,681,806. 7,654 casks of rice, foreign; 23,094 casks of rice, coastwise—valued at $700,000. 27,353,600 feet of lumber, foreign; 22,502,100 feet of lumber, coastwise—valued at $500,000. Sundries, such as wheat, flour, wool, manufactures, hides, peltries, copper ore, tallow, beeswax, drugs, &c., exported, were valued at $1,000,000. Grand total value of exports, $17,881,806. Tonnage of vessels cleared and entered, 377,876; 131,033 foreign and 246,843 coastwise.

In 1855, 178,194 bales of upland, and 6,993 bales of sea island cotton, foreign; 195,714 bales of upland, and 7,474 bales of sea island cotton, coastwise—valued at $17,766,215. 5,149 casks of rice, foreign; 3,071 casks of rice, coastwise—valued at $213,798.* 19,004,308 feet of lumber, foreign; 6,495,692 feet of lumber, coastwise—valued at $255,000.† 423,375 bushels of wheat, coastwise—

* The crop this year was nearly destroyed by the gale in September, 1854, hence the small quantity exported in this year. The scarcity, of course, increased its value, consequently the increase in value as compared with 1854.

† The yellow fever in the fall of 1854 (occurring at the time when the trade in lumber is extensive) prevented the rafting of lumber to market, hence the decrease of exports of this article, as compared with the year previous, amounting to nearly fifty per cent.

valued at $719,737. 31,632 boxes of copper ore, coastwise—valued at $474,480. Sundries—valued at $700,000. Total value of exports, $20,129,230. Tonnage of vessels cleared and entered, 510,-475; 151,136 foreign and 359,339 coastwise.

In 1856, 177,182 bales of upland, and 8,138 bales of sea island cotton, foreign; 200,426 bales of upland, and 7,346 bales of sea island cotton coastwise—valued at $19,100,000. 7,880 casks of rice, foreign; 22,027 casks of rice, coastwise—valued at $780,000. 21,500,-000 feet of lumber, foreign; 13,387,500 feet of lumber, coastwise—valued at $350,000. 325,000 bushels of wheat, coastwise—valued at $445,000. 23,500 boxes copper ore, coastwise—valued at $352,-500. Sundries—valued at $1,000,000. Total value of exports, $22,027,500. Tonnage of vessels cleared and entered, 448,780; 157,088 foreign and 291,692 coastwise.

In 1857, 152,228 bales of upland, and 6,611 bales of sea island cotton, foreign; 158,791 bales of upland, and 10,028 bales of sea island cotton, coastwise. 6,787 casks of rice, foreign; 20,749 casks of rice, coastwise. 36,752,502 feet of lumber, foreign; 7,990,568 feet of lumber, coastwise. 354,333 bushels of wheat, and 11,715 boxes of copper ore, coastwise. Total value of all of these exports, including sundries, $22,500,000.

In 1858, 159,141 bales of upland, and 8,561 bales of sea island cotton, foreign; 117,680 bales of upland, and 7,447 bales of sea island cotton, coastwise. 7,284 casks of rice, foreign; 24,061 casks of rice, coastwise. 19,611,391 feet of lumber, foreign; 8,754,265 feet of lumber, coastwise. 326,777 bushels of wheat, coastwise. 3,202 boxes of copper ore, coastwise.

In 1859, 253,743 bales of upland, and 8,298 bales of sea island cotton, foreign; 198,523 bales of upland, and 8,489 bales of sea island cotton, coastwise. 6,836 casks of rice, foreign; 31,294 casks of rice, coastwise. 29,384,315 feet of lumber, foreign; 9,543,669 feet of lumber, coastwise. 136,484 bushels of wheat.

In 1860, 307,579 bales of upland, and 6,505 bales of sea island cotton, foreign—valued at $17,210,168. 6,790 tierces of rice, foreign—valued at $148,300. 20,723,350 feet of lumber, foreign—valued at $400,151. Total value of exports to foreign ports, $17,-798,922.

In 1861, 1862, 1863, and 1864, the port was blockaded, consequently there were no exports or imports during these years, excepting what was run through the blockade, of which no account can be given.

In 1865 the exportations (the property of the Confederate States and of the citizens of Savannah) was carried on exclusively by the officers and men of the United States government in its ships. United States officers, late in December, 1864, seized all the cotton and numerous other articles (whether the property of the Confederate government or of the citizens mattered little) and shipped the cotton to New York and the other plunder to their northern homes.

In 1866, commencing July 1st and ending June 30th, 1867, 103,317 bales of upland, and 7,676 bales of sea island cotton, foreign; 140,396 bales of upland, and 6,700 bales of sea island cotton, coastwise—valued at $37,495,173. 6,060 casks of rice, coastwise—valued at $363,300. 19,660,000 feet of lumber, foreign; 15,-496,000 feet of lumber, coastwise—valued at $765,006. 87 tons of manganese (new export)—valued at $2,052. 12,393 bales of domestics—valued at $1,858,950. 1,221 bales of wool—valued at $91,575. 10,801 barrels of naval stores—valued at $129,612. Sundries, including junk—valued at $519,821. Total value of exports, $41,225,488. Tonnage of vessels cleared and entered, 820,991; 105,401 foreign and 715,590 coastwise.

In 1868, ending June 30, 256,669 bales of upland, and 6,680 bales of sea island cotton, foreign; 234,434 bales of upland, and 5,190 bales of sea island cotton, coastwise. 22,844,387 feet of lumber, foreign; 9,152,000 feet of lumber, coastwise. 4,291 casks of rice, coastwise. Value of sundries, foreign, $26,146; value of sundries, coastwise, $43,000. 9,774 bales of domestics, coastwise. 981 bales of wool, coastwise. 92,540 bushels of wheat, coastwise. 10,593 barrels of flour, coastwise. 70,646 hides, and 12,201 barrels of rosin and turpentine, coastwise. 1,132 hogsheads of clay, coastwise. 467 rolls of leather, coastwise. Total value of exports, $50,-226,209.

In 1868, for the quarter ending September 30, the value of exports were, $3,649,812; $382,602 foreign and $3,267,210 coastwise.

The following accounts of the railroad and steamship and steamboat lines will give the reader a better idea of the commercial advantages of Savannah and her future prospects than would be furnished by numberless pages of speculative articles.

THE GEORGIA CENTRAL RAILROAD.

In 1834 an experimental survey was made under the direction of Colonel Cruger, at the request and cost of the city of Savannah, to

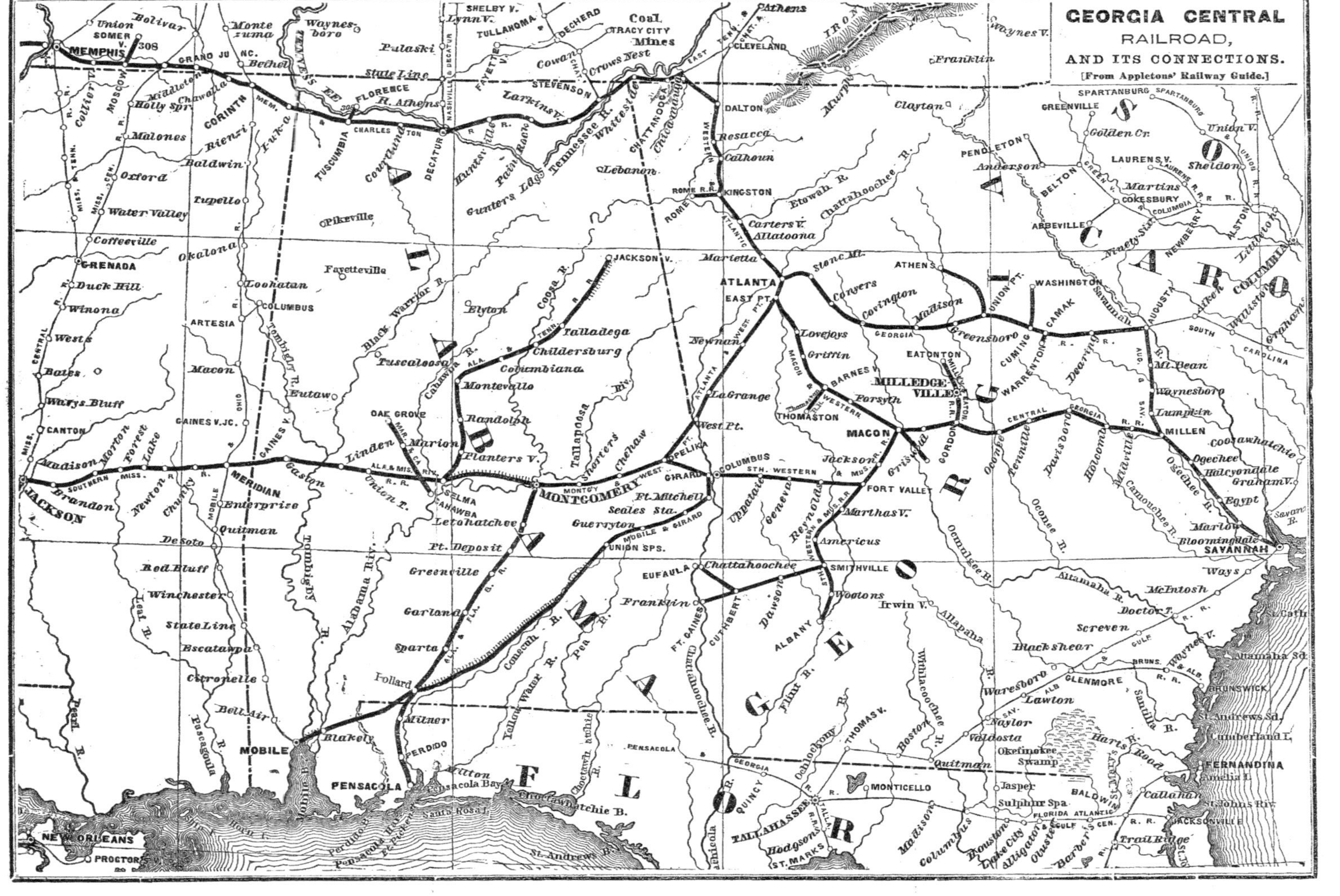
GEORGIA CENTRAL
RAILROAD,
AND ITS CONNECTIONS.
[From Appletons' Railway Guide.]
MEMPHIS
GRAND JUNC.
CORINTH
FLORENCE
TUSCUMBIA
DECATUR
STEVENSON
CHATTANOOGA
DALTON
KINGSTON
ROME
ATLANTA
EAST PT.
ATHENS
WASHINGTON
AUGUSTA
COLUMBIA
MILLEDGEVILLE
MACON
MILLEN
SAVANNAH
COLUMBUS
MONTGOMERY
SELMA
JACKSON
MERIDIAN
MOBILE
PENSACOLA
NEW ORLEANS
EUFAULA
SMITHVILLE
FORT VALLEY
THOMASTON
TALLAHASSEE
FERNANDINA
BRUNSWICK
GRENADA
CANTON
Okefinokee Swamp

ascertain the most practicable route to Macon. In 1835 the Central Railroad and Banking company of Georgia was organized, and in 1836 commenced operations. In May, 1838, sixty-seven miles were graded, and the superstructure laid twenty-six miles from the city, to which point engines were running. In July passenger trains began running regularly, at once yielding an income to the company. On the 13th of May, 1843, the track was complete to the depot in Macon, and a train passed over the whole line, one hundred and ninety miles. To the untiring zeal and administrative ability of W. W. Gordon, Esq. (the president of the road), ably assisted by Thomas Purse, Esq., is the State indebted for the completion of its greatest enterprise.

The depot of the company in Savannah is situated in the southwestern portion of the city, and, with its warehouses and machine-shops, occupies a tract of five acres of land, bestowed upon the company by the City Council of Savannah. The buildings for the accommodation and requirements of the road in Savannah are upon the most extensive scale, and second to none, in extent and completeness, in the United States. The road-track, depots, &c., outside of Savannah, were destroyed by Sherman's army, but were replaced soon after the war.

An examination of the map of Georgia and the contiguous States will show that no internal improvement could be devised for greater general benefit to the commercial world than the Georgia Central railroad, extending, as it will eventually, its iron arms to the Pacific ocean. Its present connections and ramifications are from Savannah to Macon, one hundred and ninety miles, thence by the Southwestern and Muscogee railroad to Columbus, one hundred miles, with the Columbus and Opelika railroad to Opelika, on the Montgomery and West Point railroad, twenty-eight miles, thence to Montgomery, sixty-four miles, where connections are made with steamers at all landings on the Alabama river, Mobile, and New Orleans, or by rail with the Mobile and Montgomery railroad to Mobile, one hundred and eighty-six miles, thence by steamer to New Orleans. A short line of rail between Montgomery and Selma is only needed to complete a continuous railroad line to Vicksburg, Mississippi. At Millen, seventy-nine miles from Savannah, the road connects with the Augusta and Savannah railroad to Augusta, fifty-three miles, thence with the Georgia railroad to Atlanta, one hundred and seventy-one miles, with the Western Atlantic railroad to Chattanooga, Tennessee, one hundred and thirty-eight miles, there connecting with the Georgia and East Tennessee railroad northward, through Tennessee and Virginia, to New York. The road also connects at Augusta with the South Carolina road, and passengers can have the choice of two routes through South Carolina, North Carolina, and Virginia to Washington, through Maryland, Delaware, and Pennsylvania to New York city. At Chattanooga with the Nashville and Chattanooga railroad to Stevenson, thirty-eight miles, thence by the Memphis and Charleston railroad to Memphis, Tennessee, two hundred and seventy-two miles. At Gordon, one hundred and seventy miles from Savannah, a branch of the Central railroad connects with the Milledgeville and Eatonton railroad to Eatonton, thirty-eight miles. At Macon with the Macon and Western railroad to Atlanta, one hundred and three miles, thence with the Georgia railroad northward. At Atlanta with the Atlanta and West Point railroad to West Point, eighty-seven miles, thence with the Montgomery and West Point railroad to Montgomery, eighty-eight miles, thence southward to Mobile. At Macon it also connects with the Georgia railroad to Eufaula, Alabama, one hundred and forty-three miles, there connecting with steamers on the Chattahoochee river to the Gulf of Mexico. A branch of the Southwestern railroad from Smithville to Albany, twenty-three miles, connects with steamers on the Flint river to the Chattahoochee river and Gulf of Mexico. Another branch of the Southwestern railroad extends from Cuthbert to Fort Gaines, on the Chattahoochee river, twenty miles. Again, at Macon the Central railroad connects with the Brunswick and Macon railroad to Hawkinsville, fifty miles. Another branch of the Southwestern railroad from Columbus, Georgia—the Mobile and Girard railroad—extends to Thomasville, Alabama, sixty-three miles.

The Central railroad has, as stated, a continuous line, with the exception of a short gap, to Vicksburg, which will most probably be the connecting point of the Southern Pacific route with the roads leading to the Atlantic coast. The President of the Vicksburg and Meridian railroad (which traverses the State of Mississipi due east and west, and is the link connecting on the inland route the Mississippi river with the States of Alabama, Georgia, and Florida), in his annual report, speaking of the Southern Pacific route, says that the shortest line from the Mississippi river to the Atlantic ocean is from Vicksburg to Savannah, six hundred and seventy-three miles, and if the passenger trains were run at twenty-five miles an hour, the time between these two cities would be twenty-seven hours, and for freight trains, running at twelve miles an hour, the time would be about fifty-six hours. The Montgomery and Selma connection (of forty-four miles) is now the great desideratum for at once securing to this line that valuable passenger business for points east of Selma, and we are gratified to learn that C. J. Pollard, the distinguished and able President of the Montgomery roads, has finally succeeded in making reliable arrangements for the speedy completion of the Montgomery and Selma road. That line must eventually be a portion of the main passenger route for the great travel from Texas and Louisiana, and a large portion of Mississippi, to the States of Alabama, Florida, Georgia, South and North Carolina. The Vicksburg, Shreveport, and Texas railroad starts from the west bank of the Mississippi, opposite Vicksburg. It passes through Monroe, on the Ouachita, and Shreveport, on the Red river, and has its terminus at the Texas State line, eighteen miles west of Shreveport. Monroe is seventy-five miles from Vicksburg, and Shreveport about one hundred and ninety. Previous to the war the road was built, equipped, and in successful operation between Monroe and the Vicksburg terminus, bringing on its trains a considerable amount of valuable business to Vicksburg and passengers for the Vicksburg and Meridian railroad. The road was built from Shreveport to the Texas line, eighteen miles, at which point the Southern Pacific railroad commences, and from thence runs to Marshall, in Texas. Twenty-four miles of that portion of the Southern Pacific road has already been built, equipped, and put in operation. With railroad connection established between Vicksburg and Shreveport, there would be at once a great increase of travel and trade seeking exit at Savannah, with the completion of the Montgomery and Selma road.

The time by rail from Shreveport to Vicksburg would be about ten hours; and, as a matter of economy, both in time and money, we would get all the New Orleans travel from that direction. A large amount of Texas and Louisiana cotton, of beef cattle, and also of Texas wheat—the latter forty to sixty days earlier than it is elsewhere ready for market—would be brought to Vicksburg for sale and transhipment. Then the travel from all northern, eastern, and central Texas, going to points east, northeast, and southeast from Vicksburg, would take this route and *vice versa.* Sooner or later these important eastern connections will be completed, constituting a main trunk line, stretching from the Atlantic, at Savannah, via the Southern Pacific railroad, to San Diego and San Francisco on the Pacific, and will eventually become the grand avenue of the world's travel and traffic. This route has been carefully surveyed and found to be the shortest, most eligible, and advantageous in every particular, that can be constructed between the two oceans. The shortest distance and time, on this line, from ocean to ocean, will be from San Diego to Savannah, two thousand and seventy-two miles, or one hundred and three hours railroad time, estimating the speed at twenty miles an hour. To Charleston, two thousand one hundred and eighty-four miles, one hundred and nine hours; and to Norfolk, two thousand five hundred and thirty-one miles, one hundred and twenty-six hours, railroad time.

Possessing such superior climatic advantages over the more northern route, being on a latitudinal line between the thirty-second and thirty-third degrees from Savannah to San Diego, with the additional advantage of a shorter distance, must make this the preferred route for travel and traffic between the Pacific and Atlantic seaports. The advantages which will flow from such a continental and latitudinal line can not be estimated or overestimated, and must be obvious to the most obtuse.

By the laws of trade, the transportation of merchandise, as well as people, will adopt that route which most fully combines the recommendations of speed, cheapness, safety, and comfort, and this will be the line that will most fully meet those requirements. Ship loads of teas, silks, spices, and other valuable Asiatic articles of commerce destined for Europe, will be shipped via California, and then by rail over this grand continental and always open and available line to Savannah, for reshipment to European ports—making the voyage from Canton, China, to Savannah in about twenty-three days; to New York in twenty-four days; and to London in from thirty-five to forty days, against two hundred days from Canton to New York, and about the same time from Canton to Liverpool by sea.

The completion of the Montgomery and Selma connection of forty-four miles, and about one hundred and ninety miles from Monroe, Louisiana, to Shreveport, would force the early completion of the Southern Pacific railroad, and place at once direct, expeditious, and ample steamship communications from Savannah to all the important European ports. The establishment of such a direct and speedy intercourse between the Chinese ports, Savannah, and New York, via California, would revolutionize the commerce of Europe and America with China; the southern direct lines would then be the carriers between the Atlantic and Pacific of the travel and trade from Europe to China, and from China to Europe, which now takes a voyage of months to accomplish.

The officers of the Central road are: Colonel William M. Wadley, President; Colonel J. F. Waring, Acting Master of Transportation; Colonel William M. Wadley, Andrew Low, John R. Wilder, William B. Johnston, General J. F. Gilmer, George W. Wylly, John Cunningham, Edward Padelford, and George W. Anderson, Directors.

ATLANTIC AND GULF RAILROAD.

The depot grounds of this road are in the southeastern portion of the city, fronting on Liberty and East Broad streets, and contain over eighty acres of land, well situated for the purpose and affording ample room for the future requirements of the company.

This road is the main thoroughfare connecting Savannah with Florida, southern and southwestern Georgia, and eastern Alabama. It extends to Bainbridge, on the Flint river, a distance of two hundred and thirty-seven miles. Blackshear, in Pierce county, Homersville, in Clinch county, Valdosta, in Lowndes county, Quitman, in Brooks county, and Thomasville, are all thriving centres of local trade, and are the county seats of the respective counties in which they are situated. Bainbridge, the present terminus of the road, bids fair to become a considerable town. A number of steamers are employed in the river trade, and a large part of the business of Columbus, Eufaula, and Fort Gaines, and of the country lying adjacent to the Flint, Chattahoochee, and Apalachicola rivers, passes through this place to Savannah.

The system of railroads in Florida is connected with Savannah by a branch road forty-eight miles in length, extending from Lawton, one hundred and thirty-two miles from Savannah, to Live Oak, on the Pensacola and Georgia railroad. Over this route the greater part of the produce of Florida is carried to market, and the facilities of communication which it affords have done much to bring into general notice the remarkable advantages of this delightful region, which year by year is becoming more frequented by tourists, invalids, and persons interested in the culture of tropical fruits.

Another branch road is now being located from Thomasville to Albany, fifty-seven miles, which will be the connecting link between the Southwestern and Atlantic and Gulf railroads.

The Macon and Brunswick railroad, now under construction, crosses this road at a point fifty-six miles from Savannah.

By examining the accompanying map the reader will see how large an area of country is tributary to this enterprise. A correct estimate of its value to Savannah can only be found after a knowledge of the motives which led to its construction.

The first organization was effected in 1853, under the title of the Savannah and Albany railroad. Dr. John P. Screven, who was president, until his death, of the several corporations now merged in the present company, was a prime mover in the project; to his energy and foresight the State of Georgia and the city of Savannah are in a great measure indebted for this enduring monument of their public spirit and wisdom. With the name of Dr. Screven must be joined that of Colonel Nelson Tift, the earliest projector of railroads in southwestern Georgia, and the present representative from that part of the State to the United States Congress. Messrs. John Stoddard, Hiram Roberts, William Duncan, H. D. Weed, and Dr. R. D. Arnold, who were on the Board of Directors as at first organized, are still Directors of the Atlantic and Gulf Railroad company.

In 1854 the name of the company was changed to the Savannah, Albany, and Gulf Railroad company. The immediate importance to the city of Savannah of securing the business of southern Georgia and Florida was so evident that it was determined to attain this object before completing the grand project at first intended, viz: the construction of an air line from Savannah to Pensacola or Mobile. A subscription of one million dollars was obtained from the city, and from this policy ensued the construction of the present line to Bainbridge. Many difficulties were experienced in consequence of the existence of a scheme to build a road from Brunswick through the same country. These difficulties were at length adjusted by leaving the construction of the line west of Screven station, sixty-eight miles from Savannah, to a company organized for the purpose, under the name of the Atlantic and Gulf Railroad company, for which State aid was obtained, amounting to one million dollars (the city of Savannah also subscribing two hundred thousand dollars). The Savannah, Albany, and Gulf Railroad company was consolidated with this company in 1863.

The beginning of the late war found the road completed to Thomasville, two hundred miles from Savannah, where further progress was arrested until the summer of 1867. The work was then resumed and the road opened to Bainbridge in December of that year.

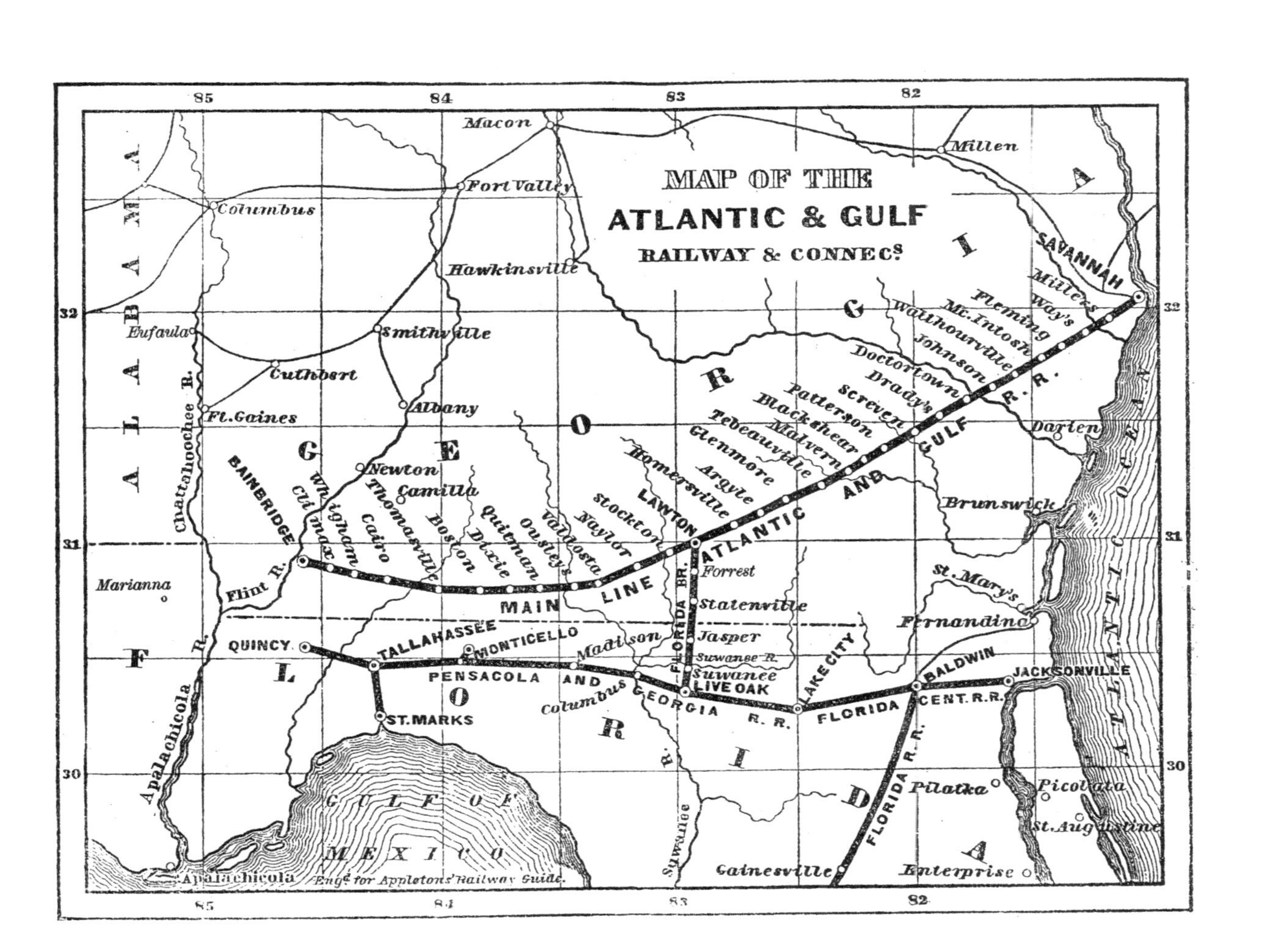

MAP OF THE
ATLANTIC & GULF
RAILWAY & CONNECS.
ALABAMA
GEORGIA
FLORIDA
GULF OF MEXICO
ATLANTIC OCEAN
Macon
Millen
Fort Valley
Columbus
Hawkinsville
SAVANNAH
Eufaula
Smithville
Cuthbert
Ft. Gaines
Albany
Newton
Camilla
BAINBRIDGE
Climax
Whigham
Cairo
Thomasville
Boston
Dixie
Quitman
Ousley's
Valdosta
Naylor
Stockton
LAWTON
Homersville
Argyle
Glenmore
Tebeauville
Malvern
Blackshear
Patterson
Screven
Dradys
Doctortown
Johnson
Walthourville
McIntosh
Fleming
Way's
Millers
ATLANTIC AND GULF R. R.
MAIN LINE
Darien
Brunswick
St. Mary's
Fernandina
Chattahoochee R.
Flint R.
Marianna
Apalachicola R.
QUINCY
TALLAHASSEE
MONTICELLO
Madison
Forrest
Statenville
Jasper
Suwanee R.
Suwanee
LIVE OAK
FLORIDA BR.
PENSACOLA AND GEORGIA R. R.
Columbus
LAKE CITY
FLORIDA R. R.
BALDWIN
CENT. R. R.
JACKSONVILLE
ST. MARKS
Suwanee R.
Pilatka
Picolata
St. Augustine
Gainesville
Enterprise
Apalachicola
Engd for Appletons' Railway Guide.
85
84
83
82
32
31
30

In these seven years the enterprise passed through many trials. The existence of war prevented the company from deriving any profit from their property, which at the collapse of the Southern Confederacy was almost a ruin. For nearly one third of the length of the road the track was torn up and the depots and bridges burned. The resources of the company thus destroyed, it was with difficulty that the work of reconstruction was commenced in October, 1865, and the road reopened for business in March, 1866. In 1866 the construction of the Florida branch was resumed and completed in October of that year.

From this brief statement the reader may judge of the future prospect of this great project—originated by a few thoughtful and public-spirited men, solely for the aggrandizement of the State of Georgia and of its metropolis, carried forward through political and financial difficulties that threatened its very existence, its property rendered useless, and its business disorganized by war and its attendant calamities, yet reviving with the return of peace, to be pressed forward with renewed vigor as the opportunity offered, never failing to serve the purpose for which it was originally intended.

Extending, as this road does, directly west from the most western Atlantic seaport, its advantages in connection with that great Southern Pacific road, which must be one day built, are obvious at the first glance upon the map.

From its Florida terminus a line through southern Florida to Tampa will furnish a practicable route to Cuba and South America, terminating as it will upon what Colonel Screven has so aptly designated as "the great wharf-head which nature has constructed between the Atlantic and the Gulf of Mexico."

The officers of this road are: John Screven, President; Henry S. Haines, General Superintendent; D. Macdonald, Treasurer.

The Board of Directors are: John Screven, Jno. Stoddard, Henry D. Weed, W. H. Wiltberger, Hiram Roberts, William Duncan, R. D. Arnold, Charles Green, E. C. Anderson, Octavus Cohen, J. L. Villalonga, J. W. Spain, A. T. McIntyre, B. F. Bruton, C. J. Munnerlyn.

THE SAVANNAH, SKIDAWAY, AND SEABOARD RAILROAD.

On the 20th of December, 1866, the General Assembly of the State of Georgia granted a charter to William R. Symons and James J. Waring, for Skidaway island; George W. Wylly and Joseph S. Claghorn, for the Isle of Hope; George M. Willett and Lemuel

Hover, for Montgomery; Alvin N. Miller and William Neyle Habersham, for White Bluff; Edward J. Purse and Herbert A. Palmer, for the city of Savannah, and such other individuals as the above-named persons shall associate with them, to incorporate the Savannah, Skidaway, and Seaboard Railroad company, for the purpose of opening a railroad communication from the city of Savannah to the adjacent sea islands. In July, 1868, the Council of Savannah passed an ordinance granting the company the privilege of constructing a railway through West Broad from Liberty to Bay, through Bay to East Broad, through East Broad to Gaston, and through Whitaker from Bay to Anderson, and through Drayton from Bay to Anderson streets.

The work of constructing the road to the islands was commenced in the summer of 1868. In a very short period the entire road, including the street railway, will be completed. In the language of the company's circular: "It may with truth be said, that no enterprise, involving so small an amount of capital, promises more beneficial results or pecuniary benefits than the Savannah, Skidaway, and Seaboard railroad.

"In the present state of the finances of our people, and especially 'those who can't get away,' a railroad to the 'salts' will afford an opportunity of reinvigorating their systems by breathing a salt atmosphere and bathing in the salt water—which luxuries can only be indulged in now by the few who are able to own vehicles or pay ten dollars per day for a hack. But when the cost is reduced to twenty-five or fifty cents a ride, the luxury is placed in the reach of every one. Our oldest and best physicians will bear us out in the opinion that there is nothing more invigorating and healthful to the human system than occasional relaxation from business and change of air, and, consequently, it is a blessing to place the means in the possession of every one to enjoy.

"All railroads develop the country through which they pass, and none more so than those like the one projected, near a city, affording the advantages to the business portion of a city and country residence combined, lessening the expense of living while increasing the comforts of life. It will place within the means of the most humble a home, and the facilities of getting to and from his business with ease and cheapness, whilst at the same time health is subserved and thrift and economy cultivated.

"This road will place within the means of our people the opportunity of successfully competing, in all branches of small manufacturing, with other sections of our country, by lessening the cost of production, which will react in favor of the city and its citizens in many ways, by affording them the productions at less cost, by affording more employment for labor, and by ease of access and less cost of transportation.

"Many persons from the interior of Georgia have been long accustomed to resort to our seacoast, during a portion of the summer months, for health and recreation. When proper establishments are erected for the accommodation of visitors, it is not unreasonable to suppose that the number of health and pleasure-seekers will be largely increased. Why should we not have a Nahant, a Cape Fear, or a Cape May near our city, in our Skidaway, our White Bluff, our Warsaw, or our Green Island?

"It is justly claimed for this road that it will be the beginning of a development which, in years to come, will spread over all the neighboring islands, making pleasant and happy homes for thousands; exempting our citizens from the so-called necessity, year after year, of paying tribute to other portions of the country."

The depot of the company will be located in Dillon Town. The officers of the company are: Colonel Joseph S. Claghorn, President; Colonel William R. Symons, Superintendent; George W. Wylly, Treasurer. The Board of Directors consists of the above-named officers, Octavus Cohen, J. W. Lathrop, Thomas Holcombe, M. Y. Henderson, A, N. Miller, and W. N. Habersham.

THE SAVANNAH AND CHARLESTON RAILROAD,

Which was destroyed during the late war, is now in course of reconstruction, and when completed will afford daily communication with Charleston and secure to Savannah a fair proportion of the products of the country through which it passes.

CANAL.

The Savannah and Ogeechee Canal company was organized as the Savannah, Ogeechee, and Altamaha Canal company about thirty years ago. The canal extends from the Savannah river to the Ogeechee river. Large quantaties of lumber and rice are annually brought to Savannah through this canal. Mr. F. Blair is president of the company.

STEAMSHIP LINES.

The blockade of the port of Savannah during the late war broke up the lines of steamship and steamboat communication from Savannah to other ports. Since the war the old lines have been re-established and new ones organized, all of which are now in successful operation.

The Macgregor line, establishing direct communication between Savannah and Liverpool, will employ ten steamships (with an average capacity each of three thousand bales of cotton), the Sarasota, Saluda, Selma, Savannah, Satilla, Waverly, Leith, Stirling, Riga, and Don. The steamships will ply regularly between Savannah and Liverpool, and will also employ a number of barks if sufficient inducements are offered. Messrs. W. M. Tunno & Co. are agents.

The Black Star line, of which Messrs. Octavus Cohen & Co. are agents, has three steamships, the Thames, Montgomery, and Huntsville, each of about twelve hundred tons burthen, which make semi-weekly trips from Savannah to New York.

The Empire line, of which Messrs. John W. Anderson's Sons & Co. are agents, has two steamships, the San Jacinto, thirteen hundred tons, and the San Salvador, nine hundred tons, which make weekly trips between Savannah and New York.

The Murray Steamship Line, of which Messrs. Hunter & Gammell are agents, has two steamships, the Leo, eight hundred and ninety tons, and the Cleopatra, one thousand and forty-five tons, which make weekly trips between Savannah and New York.

The Atlantic Mail Coast Steamship company, of which Messrs. Wilder and Fullarton are agents, has two steamships, the Herman Livingston and the General Barnes, about two thousand tons each, which make weekly trips from Savannah to New York.

The Philadelphia and Southern Mail Steamship company, of which Messrs. Hunter & Gammell are agents, has two steamships, the Wyoming, seven hundred and seventy-nine tons, and the Tonawanda, eight hundred and forty-four tons, which make weekly trips between Savannah and Philadelphia.

The Baltimore and Savannah Steamship company, of which Messrs. J. B. West & Co. are agents, has four steamships, the America, eight hundred tons, the North Point, five hundred tons, the General Custar, five hundred tons, and the Fannie, four hundred tons, which make regular trips between Savannah and Baltimore.

STEAMBOAT LINES.

The steamboat Nick King, Messrs. John W. Anderson's Sons &

Co. agents, makes weekly trips from Savannah to Palatka, touching at Brunswick, Fernandina, Jacksonville, and all intermediate points on the coast of Georgia and Florida.

The Florida and Savannah line, Messrs. Claghorn & Cunningham agents, employs one steamer, the Lizzie Baker, which makes weekly trips to Palatka, Florida, touching at all intermediate points.

The Charleston and Savannah Steam Packet line, of which Messrs. Claghorn & Cunningham are agents, employ one steamer, the Pilot Boy, which makes semi-weekly trips between Savannah and Charleston.

The Charleston, Savannah, and Florida line, of which Messrs. L. J. Guilmartin & Co. are agents, has two steamboats, the Dictator and the City Point, which make semi-weekly trips from Charleston, via Savannah, to Palatka. These steamers also touch at all intermediate points.

The Erwin & Hardee line, of which Messrs. Erwin & Hardee are agents, employs the iron steamer Charles S. Hardee, which makes regular trips to Hawkinsville and all intermediate landings, touching at Darien.

The Savannah and Augusta line, of which Mr. M. A. Cohen is agent, employs two steamers, the Katie and the Swan, which run regularly between Savannah and Augusta.

The steamer H. M. Cool, for which Mr. M. A. Cohen is agent, plys regularly between Savannah and Darien, touching at all intermediate points.

CITY GOVERNMENT.

Savannah is governed by a Mayor and twelve Aldermen, who, together, are denominated the City Council, and are chosen annually. Savannah is more fortunate than many other cities of the South, in having for her rulers men who are identified with her interests and are the choice of her citizens. The present officers are:

Mayor.—Edward C. Anderson.

Chairman of Council.—Martin J. Ford.

Aldermen.—Martin J. Ford, Henry Brigham, John L. Villalonga, Frederick W. Sims, William Hunter, Francis L. Guc, Alvin N. Miller, George W. Wylly, William H. Burroughs, James J. Waring, Mathias H. Meyer, Charles C. Millar.

Clerk of Council.—James Stewart.

City Treasurer.—John Williamson.

Assistant City Treasurer.—Magnus Lowenthal.

City Marshal.—Thomas S. Wayne.

City Surveyor.—John B. Hogg.

Clerk of City Market.—Isaac Brunner.

City Printer.—J. Holbrook Estill.

Messenger of Council.—F. J. Cercopely.

Judge of City Court.—Walter S. Chisholm.

Clerk of City Court.—Phillip M. Russell, Sr.

City Sheriff.—Charles J. White.

Corporation Attorney.—Edward J. Harden.

Jailor.—Waring Russell.

Keeper of Laurel Grove Cemetery.—A. F. Torlay.

Keeper of City Dispensary.—James Stoney.

Keeper of Forsyth Place.—Patrick Scanlan.

Keeper of Pest House.—J. J. Stokes.

Keeper of Powder Magazine.—Henry L. Davis.

Pump Contractor.—Alfred Kent.

Measurers and Inspectors of Lumber and Timber.—D. C. Bacon, A. McAlpin, John R. Tebeau, T. B. Wylly, John T. Lineberger, C. H. Weber, William H. Lyon, Z. N. Winkler, John J. Backley, A. F. Bennett, S. B. Dasher, A. B. LaRoche, J. F. O'Byrne.

Port Wardens.—Robert D. Walker, Richard T. Turner, William H. Patterson, W. W. Wash, William R. Symons.

Weighers of Hay.—J. P. Williamson, A. Goeble, Lawrence Connell, William E. Gue.

Keeper of City Clock.—F. Brown.

Chimney Contractors.—Patrick Naughton, eastern division; Theodore Meves, western division.

POLICE DEPARTMENT.

This department numbers about one hundred men, who are well disciplined and equipped. Their gallant conduct on the 3d of November, 1868, in preserving the peace, increased, if possible, the respect they had previously won. The quiet of the city tells more powerfully than words of the efficiency of the force. The officers are:

Chief.—General Robert H. Anderson.

1st Lieutenant and Chief of Detective Force.—William Wray.

1st Lieutenant.—J. T. Howard.

2d Lieutenant.—Charles H. Bell.

Sergeants.—James Foley, Martin Houlihan, John Green, James Leonard, William M. Moran, Henry Ling.

FIRE DEPARTMENT.

This department is complete and efficient in organization and well supplied with apparatus. Previous to 1824 there was no regularly organized department. The first fire in Savannah occurred in 1737, after which the townsmen preferred charges against one Mr. Jones for "standing with his hands in his pockets looking on while his townsmen were working passing buckets of water and using other methods for putting out the fire." Whether this primitive method of extinguishing fires was in vogue until 1824 cannot be accurately stated. In that year the Savannah Fire company was organized. It had several hand engines under its control, which were worked by negroes. Other companies were formed and worked by the young men of Savannah, but were subject to the control of the Savannah Fire company until the 29th of January, 1867, when the present department was organized. The first and second officers of each company of the department, and the following officers, transact all business connected with the department:

Chief.—James F. Waring.

1st Assistant Engineer.—Charles Gordon.

2d Assistant Engineer.—J. A. Roberts.

Secretary.—Charles J. White.

Treasurer.—Thomas F. Butler.

The following companies are connected with the department:

The Washington Fire company was organized on the 22d of February, 1847. The company has a first-class steamer, the Washington, and numbers about seventy members. The officers are: James A. Barron, Foreman; James Kearney, 2d Foreman; S. Harrigan, 3d Foreman; John H. Straus, 4th Foreman; C. C. Wakefield, Secretary; H. J. McDonnell, Treasurer.

The Oglethorpe Fire company was incorporated in December, 1847. The company has a third-class steamer, the John W. Anderson, and numbers one hundred and sixty members. The officers are: Philip M. Russell, President; N. Hess, 1st Foreman; Chas. F. O'Neal, 2d Foreman; J. B. Sibley, 3d Foreman; R. Wayne Russell, Secretary; C. L. Lopez, Treasurer; and Dr. R. J. Nunn, Surgeon.

The Mechanics Hook and Ladder company was organized as the Young America Fire company on the 5th of December, 1848, and under its present name since the war. The apparatus of the company is elegant and admirably adapted for its purpose. The company numbers forty members, with the following officers: Wm. D. Dixon, President; J. J. McKenzie, 1st Foreman; C. C. Blancho, 2d Foreman; H. Bogardus, Secretary; D. Ferguson, Treasurer.

The Germania Fire company was organized on the 7th of December, 1853. The company has a second-class steamer, the J. J. Waver, and a full roll. The officers are: John Schwarz, Foreman; C. Hirt, 2d Foreman; R. B. Borchert, 3d Foreman; P. Schaffer, 4th Foreman; Alfred Kolp, Secretary; M. H. Myers, Treasurer.

The Metropolitan Fire company was organized on the 21st of July, 1865. The company has a third-class steamer, the F. S. Bartow, and fifty active members. The officers are: Thomas F. Butler, President; Thomas A. Maddox, 1st Vice-President; H. M. Branch, 2d Vice-President; J. J. Abrams, Secretary; George C. Lewis, Assistant Secretary; John Fernandez, Treasurer.

The Marshall Hose company was organized on the 19th of June, 1867, and has a full roll and a full supply of hose and apparatus. The officers are: Charles J. White, President; William O. Godfrey, 1st Foreman; Alfred Robider, 2d Foreman; W. J. Tomlinson, Secretary; and Joseph Fernandez, Treasurer.

The Screven Hose company was organized on the 1st of June, 1868, and, having a full supply of hose and apparatus, is attached to the Oglethorpe company. The officers are: Isaac Russell, President; F. M. Tidwell, 1st Foreman; A. Mickler, 2d Foreman; O. B. Johnson, 3d Forman; G. E. Bevans, Secretary; W. A. Sercy, Treasurer; and Dr. T. C. Harden, Surgeon.

There are six fire companies under the control of the department worked by colored men. Four of the companies, the Pulaski, Franklin, Columbus, and Tomichichi, have hand engines, and the other two are axe companies.

The department has a neat and capacious building, located on the corner of South Broad and Abercorn streets, in which the departmental meetings are held and all business connected with the department transacted.

The Savannah Fire company is still an organized body, but has no apparatus. C. C. Casey, Chief Fireman; F. Blair, 2d Fireman; and James L. Haupt, 3d Fireman.

POPULATION.

The population of Savannah is estimated to be about forty-five thousand persons. The first regular census of the city was taken in 1810, when the population was 5,195; in 1820, 7,523; in 1830,

7,773; in 1840, 11,214; in 1850, 14,000; and at the close of the war (1865), 24,000; making the increase, within the past three years, 21,000.

EDUCATION.

The subject of education has always been of interest to the citizens of Savannah, and all measures for this purpose have met with favor. The first academy in Savannah was incorporated as the Chatham County Academy in 1788, and flourished for many years. A portion of its spacious brick building, on South Broad street, is still used for educational purposes. The first free school, known as the Savannah Free School, was established in 1816. There are at present a number of denominational and private schools.

The public school system of Savannah is equal to any, and superior to many others, in the United States. About one thousand pupils are instructed in the public schools. The Board of Education controlling these schools consists of R. D. Arnold, M. D., John Stoddard, Edward C. Anderson, Henry Williams, Solomon Cohen, John C. Ferrill, John L. Villalonga, John Williamson, Rev. D. H. Porter, James B. Read, M. D., Rev. S. Landrum, and Barnard Mallon. R. D. Arnold, M. D., President; John Stoddard, Vice-President; W. H. Baker, Secretary; John L. Villalonga, Treasurer.

The following schools, of which Mr. W. H. Baker is superintendent, are under the charge of the Board of Education. The houses are large and well located, and the school-rooms well furnished and comfortable:

Boys' High School, corner of Barnard and Taylor streets. W. H. Baker, Principal; B. M. Zettler and Miss V. Miller, Assistants.

Boys' Grammar School, corner of Barnard and Taylor streets. H. F. Train, Principal; Miss E. Frew, Assistant.

Girls' High School, corner of Abercorn and Gordon streets. B. Mallon, Principal; Miss Fannie A. Dorsett and Miss Selina J. Jones, Assistants.

Girls' Grammar School, corner of Abercorn and Gordon streets. Miss M. A. McCarter, Principal; Miss Lizzie Miller and Miss M. L. Harris, Assistants.

Intermediate School, Armory Hall, Wright square. Jos. E. Way, Principal; Miss A. M. Gould and Miss E. F. Bourquin, Assistants.

Primary School, Armory Hall, Wright square. Miss M. E. Davenport, Principal; Miss A. N. Harden and M. W. Mallard, Assistants.

Boys' Intermediate School, in the Chatham Academy building. Miss Eunice Mallery, Principal.

Girls' Grammar School, in the Chatham Academy building. Miss E. W. Carter, Principal; Professor H. Elliott, Teacher of French; Professor J. Newman, Teacher of Music.

The Catholics have two free schools, one in St. John's parish and the other in St. Patrick's parish. The school building of the former is located on the corner of Perry and Abercorn streets. About two hundred and fifty pupils attend this school, of which Mr. O'Brien is Principal; Miss A. Robinson and Miss K. McCluskey, Assistants.

The school of St. Patrick's parish is located in the rear of St. Patrick's church, near the Central Railroad depot. There are about one hundred and seventy-five scholars attending this school, of which Mr. Edward McCort is Principal; Mr. Luke Logan and Miss B. Kirk, Assistants.

Savannah Hebrew Collegiate Institute. Of all the educational establishments which grace our "Forest City," none stands higher or claims more admiration than this noble institution. Although it is in its infancy, it has already given the most unmistakable proofs of the immense advantages it is destined to confer upon the citizens of Savannah, if not indeed upon the people of Georgia. Claiming to be of Hebrew origin, and therefore bearing its present name, it has, notwithstanding, thrown its doors open to every sect and creed, and, knowing no distinction of faith, it receives children of every denomination within its walls, and, regarding them only as children of the Universal Father, it labors to inculcate in their minds those sublime principles of general religion in which all mankind agree, while at the same time it confers upon them the greatest of all earthly treasures—a thorough and practical education. Organized for the purpose of advancing the interests of Savannah and enlarging her educational facilities, it very praiseworthily knows no difference between the rich and the poor, but, making respectability its only condition, it admits children of the humbler class and educates them free of charge. The history of the institute, although brief, is very interesting. On the 22d of May, 1867, a meeting of Israelites, convened by the Rev. R. D'C. Lewin, and presided over by Octavus Cohen, Esq., took place in the synagogue of the "Mickva Israel" congregation. At this meeting the Rev. R. D'C. Lewin submitted his plans and enlisted the full co-operation of the majority of his coreligionists in Savannah.

The project being cordially approved of, Messrs. B. Phillips, A. J. Brady, S. Gertsman, A. Epstein, P. Dzialynski, W. Barnett, and Rev. R. D'C. Lewin, were elected a provisional council for the purpose of preparing the constitution and by-laws, to be submitted at a subsequent meeting. This council, having chosen as its president the Rev. Mr. Lewin, entered with spirit into the work, and on the 28th of May presented to the adjourned meeting the constitution and by-laws, which met with general approval. The preliminary steps having thus been taken, the provisional council received authority "to take charge of all further business connected with the institute until such time as the permanent council was elected."

The labors of the provisional council now commenced. As yet everything was but in embryo, while the institute itself could hardly be said to be more than an idea. The idea, however, had to become a reality, and no pains were spared by the council to effect this happy consummation of the hopes of the founder. By dint of untiring perseverance and unwearied exertions, all the many difficulties which at first impeded the progress of the enterprise were overcome. To understand fully the difficulties of the enterprise would require a perfect knowledge of the plans of the founder, which were laid out on a gigantic scale. For, while it was hoped to establish the institute upon the system pursued by European colleges, a very heavy outlay for professors became inevitable. To meet this expenditure a large number of children was needed, but as one of the essential objects in the very formation of the institute was to give gratuitous education to children whose parents were unable to pay the regular tuition fees, and as a very large number of paying pupils could hardly be expected at the commencement, the council was compelled to have recourse to private aid and to solicit donations from the Jewish public of Savannah. The appeal was readily responded to, and the Rev. Mr. Lewin, in order to facilitate the enterprise, offered his services as the gratuitous superintendent, thereby releasing the institute from the payment of a large salary. Thus, at a general meeting of the members, held on the 27th of October, the provisional council had the gratification of reporting that everything was in readiness to open the institute on the 1st of November. The first permanent council was then elected, consisting of Messrs. Octavus Cohen, B. Phillips, A. B. Weslow, H. Meinhard, M. Selig, P. Dzialynski, and S. H. Eckman, the officers being Octavus Cohen, Esq., president; A. B. Weslow, Treasurer; and B. Phillips, Secretary. On the 1st of November, the institute was opened with a professorial staff of the highest rank, and a goodly number of pupils to receive its numerous benefits.

Among the advantages offered by the institute was the delivery of public lectures, for the amusement and instruction of the public. The first course, however, through unavoidable circumstances, consisted of only two lectures; but the pleasant evenings passed in listening to the eloquent addresses of the Hon. Henry R. Jackson and the Hon. Henry S. Fitch, will not be easily forgotten.

Thus, while engaged in the most noble of human employments—the culture of the mind—the first scholastic year passed pleasantly away and the summer vacation brought the labors of the professors to a close.

For the second year ample preparations were made to render the institute still more useful to the public. The fees for tuition were reduced, additional privileges bestowed upon members, and higher studies introduced, so that on the 1st of October, 1868, the institute again set forward on its mission of education, with bright hopes for its future success. On the 27th of October, 1868, the annual meeting of members took place, and the new council was elected, as follows: Hon. Solomon Cohen, Octavus Cohen, Barnet Phillips, Simon Gertsman, Marcus Selig, Henry Meinhard, and S. H. Eckman, the officers being Hon. Solomon Cohen, President; Barnet Phillips, Secretary; and Simon Gertsman, Treasurer. By resolution of the general meeting, the Rev. R. D'C. Lewin, who during the previous year had occupied an *ex-officio* seat at the council, was declared to be a life member of that body, with right to vote on all matters appertaining to the institute.

The institute embraces: 1st, a high school for boys; 2d, an academy for girls. In both departments there are classes and divisions according to the abilities of the pupils, the studies pursued in these classes being regulated according to the respective grades.

The branches taught, in addition to the general branches pursued in schools, are geometry, algebra, book-keeping, natural philosophy, together with the French, German, Hebrew, and Latin languages.

The faculty comprises the following: Rev. R. D'C. Lewin, Superintendent and Principal of the Theological department; Charles N. West, Teacher of Belles-Lettres and Mathematics; Prof. Adolph Eiswald, Teacher of Languages; Rev. E. Fischer, Teacher of Hebrew and Theology; Edwin Knapp, Teacher of Book-keeping.

AMUSEMENTS.

The love of amusement is strong among the citizens of Savannah, which is evinced by the numerous rifle, boat, and other clubs, in the sports of which old and young engage with the keenest zest.

The THEATRE, situated on the east side of Chippewa square, is the first and most prominent among the places of amusement. It enjoys the reputation of being the best adapted for its purpose of any between Baltimore and New Orleans.

ST. ANDREW'S HALL is a large brick building, situated on the south side of Broughton at the corner of Jefferson street. The

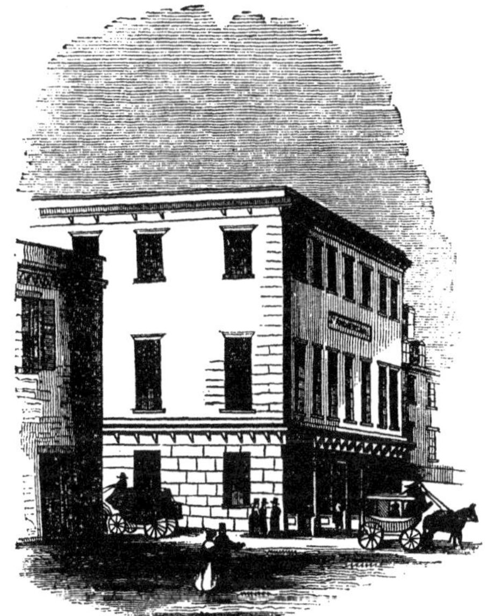

ST. ANDREW'S HALL.

hall was erected and owned by the St. Andrew's society of Savannah, but was sold to Mr. David R. Dillon during the late war. It is capacious, and complete in its arrangements for the comfort and convenience of audiences.

The MUSEUM, situated on the northeast corner of Bull and Taylor streets, is well kept, and an hour or two can be delightfully spent among the rare curiosities there on exhibition.

PUBLIC AND SOCIETY BUILDINGS.

There are a large number of fine public and society buildings in Savannah, among them the Exchange, Central Railroad Bank, State Bank, Custom House, Hall of the Georgia Historical Society, Medical College, Abrahm's Home, Female Asylum, Masonic Hall, and the three prominent hotels, the Pulaski House, Screven House, and Marshall House.

The EXCHANGE was built in 1799 by a joint-stock company, in which the city was a stockholder to the amount of twenty-five shares. The ground was leased to the company for ninety-nine years. The cost of erection was twenty thousand dollars. The city purchased stock from the inception of the company until 1812, when the building came into the possession of the city, and has since been used as a City Hall. A few years since it was enlarged to its present dimensions. The Mayor's court-room—in which the City Council also meets—the offices of the Mayor, Clerk of Council, City Treasurer, Surveyor, and Marshall, are in the upper portion of the building. The lower stories, one on a line with the top of the bluff and two beneath, are used as offices by private parties.

The GEORGIA HISTORICAL SOCIETY, upon the petition of Hon. J. M. Berrien, Hon. James M. Wayne, Hon. M. H. McAllister, I. K. Tift, Right Rev. William Bacon Stevens, George W. Hunter, Henry K. Preston, Colonel William Thorne Williams, Judge Chas. S. Henry, Judge John C. Nicoll, Judge William Law, Judge Robert M. Charlton, Dr. Richard D. Arnold, and A. A. Smets, was chartered by the legislature in 1839, "for the purpose of collecting, preserving, and diffusing information relating to the State of Georgia in particular, and of American history generally." The society was formed and a building erected on Bryan street. It is a beautiful edifice, and admirably adapted for the purpose. The society has published several valuable works. There are at present in the library seven thousand five hundred volumes, among them many rare books. There are also a large number of valuable manuscripts. There is, in connection with the society, a Scientific section, the object of which is to investigate and discuss practical questions and subjects in chemistry, mechanics, and kindred branches. The society numbers two hundred members, with the following officers: Hon. E. J. Harden, President; Dr. W. M. Charters, 1st Vice-President; Gen. A. R. Lawton, 2d Vice-President; Dr. R. D. Arnold, Corresponding Secretary; Dr. Easton Yonge, Recording Secretary; W. S. Bogart,

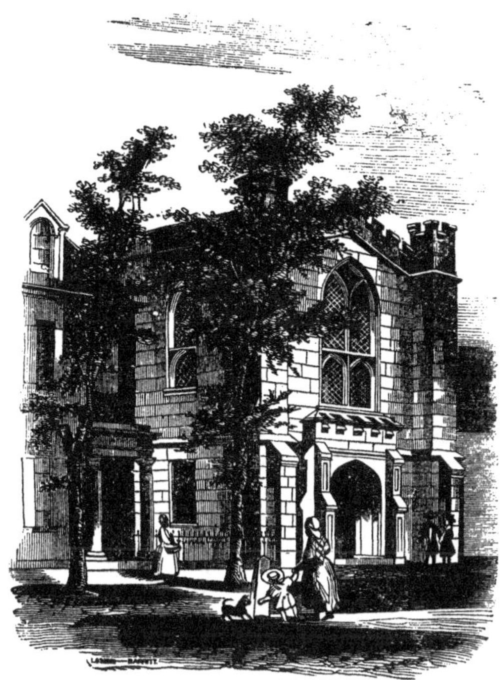

GEORGIA HISTORICAL SOCIETY.

Treasurer; J. S. F. Lancaster, Librarian; W. T. Williams, W. B. Hodgson, H. R. Jackson, William Duncan, B. Phillips, Juriah Harris, T. M. Norwood, Curators.

The Presidents of the society, since its organization, are: Hon. J. M. Berrien, Hon. James M. Wayne, Right Rev. Bishop Stephen Elliott, John Stoddard, and Hon. E. J. Harden.

The Water Works are located in the outer portion of the city, on the western side of the Ogeechee canal, close to the river, and were erected in 1853, but were not in full operation until 1854. The receiving reservoir is divided into four compartments, each about one hundred and fifty feet square and eight feet deep, so that while the clarified water from one compartment is being pumped into the city the water in the other basins is in a state of repose and becoming clear. These basins, which are capable of containing six hundred tons of water, and can be kept full, no matter how great the demand may be, are filled from the river by means of a canal with gateways into each basin. The forcing pumps are three in number, of Worthington & Baker's direct-action patent. From these the water is forced through two separate lines of pipes to the distributing reservoir. Each of the three engines is capable of delivering into the distributing reservoir one million gallons of water in twelve hours. The engines, pumps, boilers, and lines of pipe are duplicated, and a failure of a full supply of water at all times is almost impossible.

The distributing reservoir is located in Franklin square, about a half-mile distant from the receiving reservoir. It is a circular iron tank, thirty feet in diameter and twenty-five feet high, placed upon a massive structure of brick, thirty-five feet in diameter at the bottom and thirty feet at the top. A hollow shaft of brick work is carried up in the centre to the full height. Resting upon the inner and outer walls are cast-iron girders forming the floor upon which the wrought-iron tank rests. The bottom is on an elevation of fifty feet above the grade of the city at the Exchange. The whole height to which the water is raised by the pumps is one hundred and twenty feet.

Mr. R. H. Guerard is the Superintendent of the works, and Messrs. James Holland and William A. Luddington Engineers.

The Court-House, an edifice of brick and stucco, two stories in height, was erected in 1833. It is situated on the east side of Wright (formerly Percival) square, more generally known as Court-House square, on which all public out-door demonstrations are held. The first court-house was erected at the northeast corner of Bull street and Bay lane. A short time previous to the Revolutionary war a large brick court-house was built on the site of the present building, and was considerably injured by the British troops quartered therein, and also by the shells thrown from the American and French batteries during the siege in 1779. After the war it was repaired and devoted to its legitimate uses until 1831, when it was torn down.

The Superior court, Judge Schley, and the City court, Judge Walter S. Chisholm, hold their regular sessions in the upper story. The lower story is used for the offices of the Judges, Clerks, Ordinary, Sheriffs of the city and county, and the Receivers and Collectors of Taxes.

The POOR-HOUSE AND HOSPITAL was incorporated in 1835, upon the application of Joseph Cumming, S. C. Dunning, R. King, John Gardner, Mathew Hopkins, William R. Waring, Charles S. Henry, S. D. Corbett, Samuel Philbrick, N. G. Beard, Francis Sorrell, R. D. Arnold, and P. M. Kollock. The present commodious structure, located on Gaston, between Drayton and Abercorn streets, was erected by private subscription in 1819, and used for several years altogether as a hospital for sailors. In 1830 $18,000 was left to the

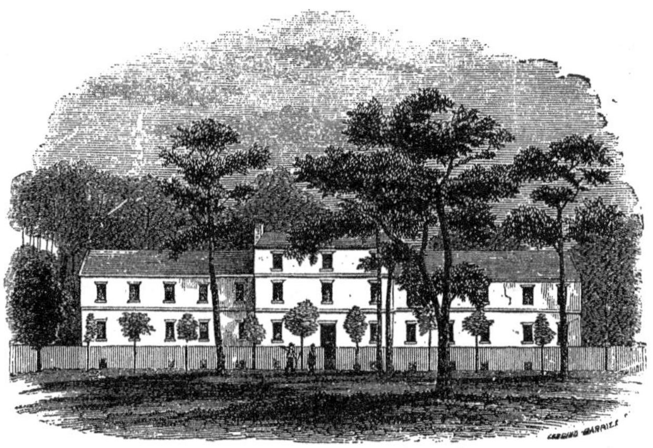

SAVANNAH POOR-HOUSE AND HOSPITAL.

institution by Messrs. James Wallace and Thomas Young. The institution is well supported by the hospital fund, the donations of fees by the attending physicians, and the State tax upon auctioneers. The officers are: Dr. William Duncan, President; Dr. R. D. Arnold, Attending Physician; Dr. W. G. Bulloch, Surgeon; Dr. Wm. Duncan, medical officer to female ward.

The ABRAHM'S HOME. On the 8th of April, 1822, a society was organized by a number of ladies of Savannah for the relief of poor widows with or without children, and destitute families generally in the city. A number of frame tenements, on South Broad street, were and are used by the society as houses for the destitute families. A few years since Mrs. Theodora Abrahms bequeathed a sum of money to be used in building an edifice to be made a home for destitute families. With the money thus contributed, the present Abrahm's Home, situated on the northwest corner of

Broughton and East Broad streets, was erected. It is a large and elegant edifice, admirably adapted for its purpose, and is under the control of the society organized in 1822. A number of aged and indigent females find shelter and comfort in this building.

The officers of the society are: Mrs. J. J. Jackson, 1st Directress; Mrs. J. H. Burroughs, 2d Directress; Mrs. Wallace Cumming, Secretary; Miss S. C. Tuffts, Treasurer.

The Bank of the State of Georgia is an imposing building. It is located on the eastern side of Johnson square. This bank,

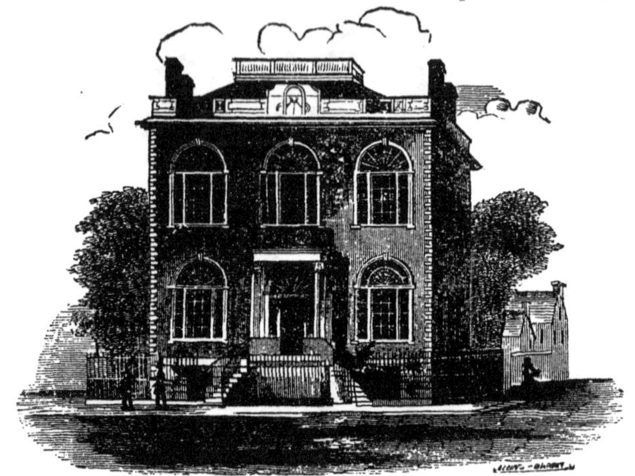

BANK OF THE STATE OF GEORGIA.

with the Merchants and Planters, Farmers and Mechanics, Planters, Marine, Bank of Commerce, and the Bank of Savannah, all in successful operation previous to and during the war, was compelled to suspend operations after the collapse of the Confederacy.

The banks in Savannah now are: The Central Railroad bank, the Savannah National bank, and the Merchants' National bank.

The Medical College, located at the northwest corner of Taylor and Habersham streets, is a fine edifice, which, for solidity, commodiousness, and perfect adaptability for all the purposes of a medical college, challenges a comparison with the best buildings of the kind in the country, and surpasses a large majority of them.

A charter to establish a medical college in Savannah was granted in 1838, but no active measures were taken to erect a building until 1852, when the late J. Gordon Howard, M. D., took the initiatory steps to that end, and Drs. P. M. Kollock, R. D. Arnold, W. G. Bulloch, C. W. West, H. L. Byrd, E. H. Martin, J. Gordon Howard, and J. B. Read petitioned the Trustees to organize them as a Faculty, they pledging themselves to erect a suitable building and to provide all apparatus necessary for instruction and illustration. The charter was not granted, owing to the opposition of a number of medical gentlemen. Nothing daunted, the gentlemen associated themselves together as a corporation under the name and style of the Savannah Medical Institute, and erected the present building, the corner-stone of which was laid on the 17th of

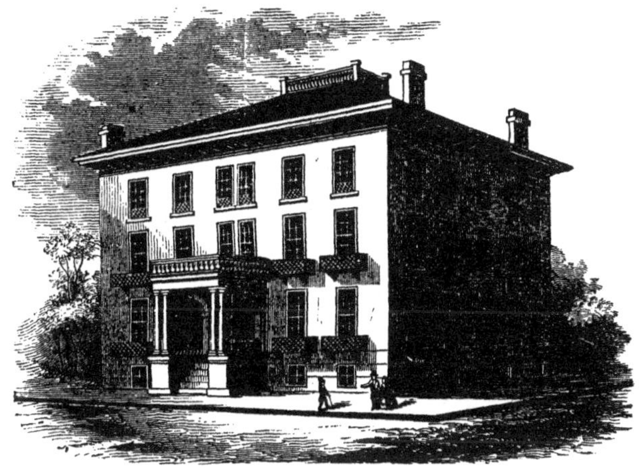

SAVANNAH MEDICAL COLLEGE.

January, 1853, by Dr. R. D. Arnold, in his capacity as Master of a Lodge of Free Masons. The following November the first course of lectures was commenced. After the capture of the city by Sherman's troops the building was used as a United States hospital, from which the United States medical officers carried off the fine apparatus, the valuable collections of minerals, the engravings and paintings for illustration, the anatomical proportions, and pathological specimens.

The members of the Faculty are: Drs. R. D. Arnold, Practice of Medicine; William G. Bulloch, Surgery; W. M. Charters, Chemistry; Juriah Harris, Physiology; P. M. Kollock, Obstetrics; J. B. Read, Materia Medica; W. R. Waring, Anatomy; William Duncan and Robert P. Myers, Demonstrators; Thomas Smith, adjunct to P. M. Kollock; Thomas J. Charlton, adjunct to W. G. Bulloch; J. G. Thomas, adjunct to Juriah Harris; J. R. Nunn, adjunct to James B. Read; W. H. Elliott, adjunct to W. M. Charters.

The officers of the Faculty are: Juriah Harris, President; W. R. Waring, Dean; P. M. Kollock, Treasurer; Robt. P. Myers, Curator.

CHATHAM COUNTY JAIL, situated in the southern part of the city, is neatly built of brick and stuccoed, and is capable of containing about one hundred prisoners. It was erected in 1845, and is under the management of Waring Russell, Esq. The first jail was situated at the northwest corner of Bay lane and Bull street, which rotted down, as did five others on the same site. Another building was erected near the site of the present court-house before the Revolutionary war, and after the war it was torn down and another built on the site occupied by Mr. A. Low's house. It was used until the present jail was built, when it was torn down to make room for dwelling-houses. In former times persons were confined for debt. They were not always actually locked up, but were permitted, upon giving sufficient surety, to go at large within "jail bounds," a certain distance each way from the jail. Should they, on any pretence or by any accident, go beyond these limits, their sureties became liable, and they themselves would be locked up. These bounds were designated at suitable intervals by small stones, like the foot-stone of a grave, with the letters "J. B." cut on them.*

Some years since a gentleman from the North, on a visit to Savannah, was walking out with a resident, when his attention was attracted by one of these stones. "What is that?" said he, "it looks as if it might have come from a graveyard."

The citizen mischievously told him that it stood at the grave of one James Benton, an old settler, indeed one of the first in the time of Oglethorpe. He went on to relate to his wondering friend how this old man (an entirely fictitious character), being a very eccentric genius, desired to perpetuate his odd whims, even after his death, and therefore left directions for his interment in one of the public squares, specifying the minutest details, even to the size and style of the stone; also binding his executors and the town authorities, in consideration of certain valuable tracts of land which he donated them, never to remove his body nor make any attempt to preserve the grave from being trampled upon, only keeping the stone up.

---

* In one or two of the squares these stones are still to be seen.

Much more of the same language did the citizen pour into the willing ears of the northerner, relating it with a minuteness of detail and a gravity of countenance which completely deceived the descendant of the Pilgrim fathers. On his return home he published in the village newspaper most wonderful accounts of the habits, manners, and customs of the people of the "Forest City."

The CUSTOM HOUSE, a noble fire-proof structure, is built of Quincy granite, and is one hundred and ten feet in length and fifty-two feet deep. It is of three stories, the first used as the post office, the second devoted to custom house purposes, and the third or upper story for United States Court room, with the usual offices.

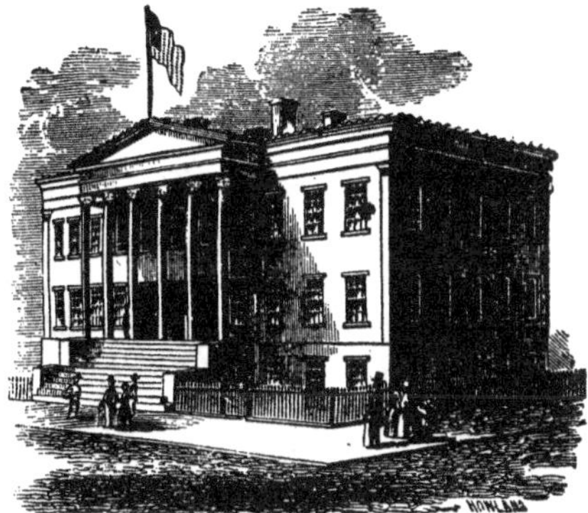

CUSTOM HOUSE.

No record remains to point out to the curious the location of the first house of customs, although there was such a one here in 1763. In 1789 Commerce row, west of the exchange, was built and the custom house established therein, wherein its duties were transacted. The customs were then removed to a building on the site now occupied by the Georgia Historical society, and afterward to the Exchange. In 1850 the present building was erected, and the customs were finally firmly located.

The FEMALE ASYLUM of Savannah had a common origin with the Union Society (which was formed in the year 1750) for the care and education of orphan and destitute children in general, who, without distinction of sex, enjoyed the benefits of its charitable appropriations until the 17th of December, 1801, at which period, for the greater benefit of both classes of children, and with a view to those more extensive results which true charity ever aims to secure, it was suggested by the Rev. Henry Holcombe, then resident pastor of the Baptist church of Savannah, to several ladies of piety and benevolence the propriety of a separation. The suggestion was approved and actively carried into effect, and the female asylum, in the year 1801, commenced a distinct and separate existence, under a Board of Directors composed of fourteen ladies, whose names are subjoined: Mrs. Elizabeth Smith, Mrs. Ann Clay, Mrs. Jane Smith; Mrs. Sarah Lamb, Secretary; Mrs. Margaret Hunter, Treasurer; Lady Ann Houston, Mrs. Holcombe, Mrs. Hannah McAllister, Mrs. Susannah Jenkins, Mrs. Ann Moore, Mrs. Moore, Mrs. Rebecca Newel, Mrs. Mary Wall, Miss Martha Stephens, Trustees, or Managers; Mrs. Lydia Myers, Matron. In

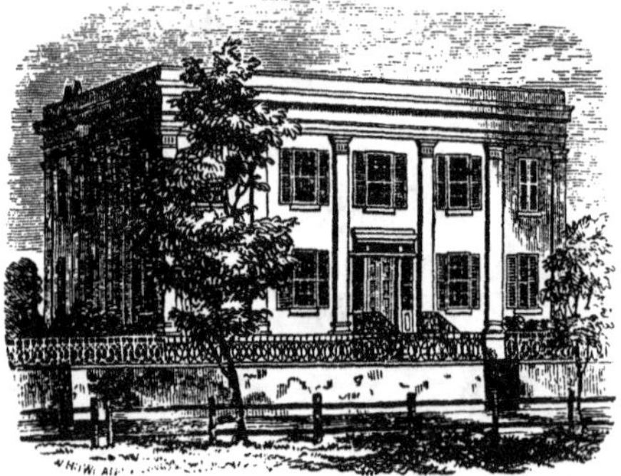

FEMALE ORPHAN ASYLUM.

1810 the legislature of Georgia granted an act of incorporation, founded on a system of rules for the better government of the institute. In 1838 (past experience having proved the necessity for a larger building and more desirable location than the one occupied in the eastern part of the city; but the limited funds of the society, at the time, prevented so desirable a change), Mrs. M. Marshall and Mrs. M. Richardsone volunteered to assist the endeavors of the Board of Managers to increase, by a public collection, the available means of the society in the accomplishment of so laudable an object. Their combined efforts happily proved successful, and the erection of the present handsome and commodious edifice on the corner of Bull and Charlton streets was the result.

The officers of the society are: Mrs. E. C. Anderson, 1st Directress; Mrs. Landrum, 2d Directress; Miss Welman, Secretary; Mrs. C. A. Lamar, Treasurer.

MONUMENTS.

The visit of General Lafayette to Savannah in 1825 was made the occasion of laying the corner-stones of two monuments to be erected, one to the memory of Gen. Nathaniel Greene and the other to the memory of Brigadier-General Count Pulaski. A committee was appointed, and under their arrangements the corner-stone of a monument to Greene was laid in Johnson square, and one to Pulaski in Chippewa square, on the 21st of March, 1825, by General Lafayette and the Masonic lodges.

Subsequently, donations were received from the citizens and others by the committee, for their erection, and in November, 1826, a lottery was granted by the legislature, for the purpose of raising the sum of $35,000, to be appropriated to the object. After a few years, the funds not having reached an amount adequate for the erection of both, it was determined to erect one only for the present; that was placed in Johnson square in 1829, and was called the "Greene and Pulaski Monument." The monument, as seen by the accompanying lithograph, is plain and without inscription. It is about fifty feet high. The lottery continued its operations and produced an amount sufficient, with other contributions, to erect

The PULASKI MONUMENT. This marble memorial to Count Casimir Pulaski, who sealed his devotion to the cause of American liberty with his blood, is situated in Monterey square. The corner-stone was laid on the 11th of October, 1853. The military, under command of Colonel A. R. Lawton, the various Masonic lodges, and a large concourse of citizens, were present during the ceremonies.

The monument is about fifty feet in height, surmounted by a statue of Liberty holding the banner of the "stars and stripes." It is perceived, at a glance, that the monument is intended for a soldier who is losing his life while fighting; wounded, he falls from his horse, still grasping his sword. The date of the event, October 9th, 1779, is recorded above the subject. The coat of arms of Poland and Georgia, surrounded by branches of laurel, ornament the cornice on two sides, or fronts; while the eagle, emblem of liberty, courage, and independence, and the symbolic bird of Poland and America, rests upon both. The cannon reversed on the corners of the die are emblematical of military loss and mourning, and give the monument a strong military character. The corner-stone laid in Chippewa square in 1825 was removed in 1853 and placed alongside of the corner-stone of the present monument.

CHURCHES.

The number and beauty of the churches of Savannah elicit the admiration of all who visit the city.

The Episcopal church was established in Savannah by Reverend Henry Herbert, D. D., in 1733, he having come over with the first settlers. Services were held in Oglethorpe's tent, or in open air, as the weather permitted, until late in that year, when a court-house was erected on Bull street at what is now the northeast corner of Bay lane, in which services were held until 1750.

Christ Church. The lot upon which this church now stands was laid out for an Episcopal church on the 7th of July, 1733, but no attempt was made to build upon it until the 11th of June 1740, when a frame building was commenced. Six years afterward the shingles were placed upon it, and it was finally completed in 1750, on the 7th of July of which year it was dedicated to the worship of God. The fire of 1796 reduced it to ashes. It was rebuilt, and was very much damaged by the gale in 1804. The present church, constructed after the Grecian Ionic order of architecture, is one of the most magnificent churches in the city. It was completed in 1838. The church records show that the following named ministers have been in charge at this church: Rev. Dr. Henry Herbert was the first. He was succeeded by Rev. S. Quincy, who remained until 1735, when Rev. John Wesley became rector. The latter was followed by the Rev. William Norris, who resided alternately in Savannah and at Frederica. Rev. Wm. Metcalf, who was appointed next, died before he entered upon his duties, and his place was filled by Rev. Mr. Orton, who died in 1742. About this period Rev. George Whitfield was in charge. Rev. T. Bosomworth, his successor, was displaced, and Rev. Mr. Zouberbuhler was appointed. He remained in charge until 1763. In 1768, 1771, and 1772, Rev. Mr. Frink was in charge. There is no record to show who were the rectors in charge from 1763 to 1768 and from 1773 to 1810, and from 1814 to 1820. From 1810 to 1814, when the church was rebuilt, Rev. John V. Bartow was in charge. Rev. Mr. Cranston became rector in 1820, and was succeeded by Rev. A. Carter, who died in 1827. He was followed by Rev. Dr. Edward Neufville, who died in 1851, having filled his responsible position for nearly a quarter of a century. He was succeeded by Rev. A. B. Carter, who remained only a short time, and Right Rev. Bishop Stephen Elliott, Bishop of the Diocese, became pastor. He resigned the charge of the church, temporarily, in November, 1859, and Rev. Dr. J. Easter was temporarily in charge, until the arrival of Rev. Dr. Batch, in February, 1860. In 1861 Bishop Elliott resumed rectorship, and Rev. Chas. H. Coley was called to assist him. Bishop Elliott died on the 21st of December, 1866. Rev. Mr. Coley remained in charge until the fall of 1868, when he received a call to the West. The church was temporarily supplied for several months by Rev. Dr. Easter, when the present rector, Rev. J. M. Mitchell, was called to the rectorship. The membership of the church is about three hundred and seventy. The Sunday-school of this church has about two hundred scholars—Dr. W. H. Elliott, Superintendent.

St. John's Church. St. John's parish was organized in 1840, and services were held in a building on South Broad west of Barnard street. The present building, built in the English style of Gothic, which prevailed in England from the year 1200 to the year 1300 of the Christian era, is located on the west side of Madison square, and was completed in 1853 and dedicated by the Right Rev. Bishop Elliott. There are about two hundred and thirty communicants in this church. The Sunday-school, with about one hundred and sixty pupils and twenty teachers, is under the superintendence of J. S. F. Lancaster.

The Church Wardens and Vestry are: W. S. Bogart and J. R. Johnson, Wardens; William Battersby, Dr. J. A. Wragg, Henry Brigham, Levi DeWitt, John M. Guerard, Edward J. Purse, John L. Villalonga, and William Tison.

The following Rectors have been in charge of the parish since its organization: Revs. Rufus M. White, George H. Clarke, C. F. McRae, and Samuel Benedict, the present rector.

Congregation "Mickva Israel." The early history of this congregation is so involved in doubt that, after the greatest possible labor and research on the part of the writer of this sketch, the task of ascertaining the exact date of organization was compelled to be abandoned. It is certain, however, that several Jews arrived from England in the year 1733, and that these brought with them two scrolls of the Law and the Ark, or receptacle for the same.

From this fact, it is reasonable to conclude that a congregation was established shortly afterward. Tradition honors a room in the neighborhood of Bay Street lane as the place in which the Hebrews first assembled for the purpose of divine worship. Then, at a later date, this temporary Synagogue was changed to a one-story wooden building on Broughton Street lane. Tradition also states that after some years a schism took place among the members of this small congregation, and doubtless this must have occurred, since the earliest manuscript extant, bearing date September 7th, 1762, is a deed of gift of a parcel of land by Mr. Sheftall to *all persons professing to be Jews*, to be used by them either as a burying-ground or as the site of a synagogue. Now this deed does not allude at all to a congregation. If, therefore, the "Mickva Israel" existed prior to this date, the tradition of a schism must be correct, and the donor of this piece of land must have purposely omitted the name of the congregation. Again, tradition asserts that this schism was subsequently healed, and the congregation reunited. Whatever may have been the real occurrences which marked the early history of the congregation, it is quite certain that it existed under its present name in the year 1790, for the old minute book, now in the possession of the congregation, contains entries as far back as that year, and the charter of the congregation bears date November 30th, 1790, during the administration of Governor Edward Telfair.

The congregation, although organized and chartered, had as yet no regular edifice for public worship, and it was not until 1815 that the first Synagogue was erected on the site of the present building, at the northeast corner of Liberty and Whitaker streets. The lot was granted by the City Council for the purpose, and the building itself was only constructed of wood, and was of small dimensions. In 1832–3 this building was destroyed by fire, but fortunately, it having been insured to the amount of $1500, the congregation was enabled to erect the present building, the difference of outlay between the amount received from the insurance and the actual cost of the new building being obtained by contributions. With all this, however, the congregation continued to remain small in numbers, which is to be attributed to the fact that no clergyman was engaged to perform divine worship, and the severe laws of the congregation prevented foreign Jews from becoming members. Time, however, cured all evils, and as soon as these restrictions, which impeded the progress of the congregation, were removed, a new life was infused into it. Thus, in the year 1852, the names of several foreigners were to be found on the list of members, and the first regular minister was appointed, after the "Mickva Israels" had been in existence over one hundred and twenty years. The Rev. Jacob Rosenfeld was the first incumbent, but in 1861 he resigned, and the congregation again continued to be without the services of a minister. This state of things continued during the war, services, however, being performed by a lay-reader.

In January, 1867, Abraham Einstein, Esq., was called to the presidential chair, and upon assuming the duties of his office he brought into the congregation about thirty new members. The want of a minister was then for the first time severely felt, and steps were at once taken to secure one. A correspondence was opened with the Rev. R. D'C. Lewin, minister of a congregation in Shreveport, La., and the position in the "Mickva Israel" was tendered to him by the Adjunta of that body. The Rev. Mr. Lewin accepted, and arrived in Savannah in March, 1867. Since that time many changes have taken place in the congregation, foremost among which have been the changes produced in synagogue worship and in the forms of the Jewish religion—the Rev. Mr. Lewin being a liberalist, and a progressionist, and belonging to that school of Judaism popularly denominated the reform school.

The "Mickva Israel" numbers about fifty members, and if the government of the congregation continues to be conducted in the same spirit as it is at present, it must undoubtedly be among the most prosperous in the country.

Congregation "B'nai Berith Jacob." This congregation was founded in September, 1860, after the departure of the Rev. J. Rosenfeld from the "Mickva Israel" congregation. It owes its origin to a society bearing the name of B'nai Berith, which existed prior to the formation of the congregation, but which resolved itself into the congregation, retaining the original name with the addition of the title "Jacob." In 1861 it was chartered, and commenced from that time worshipping in Armory Hall. The first president was Mr. Rosenfeld, who also officiated gratuitously as minister until August, 1865, when, leaving Savannah to do business in Tallahassee, Florida, Mr. Simon Gertsman commenced officiating as lay reader gratuitously. In January, 1867, this gentleman was elected president, from which date he commenced active measures to encourage the congregation by endeavoring to have a permanent building erected as a place of worship. By dint of great energy and perseverance, and after many trials and obstacles, he succeeded in his praiseworthy designs, and on the 16th of July of the same year the corner-stone of the building was laid by the Rev. R. D'C. Lewin with all the ceremonies and pomp attendant on such occasions. The work of building progressed so rapidly, under the management of the architects, Messrs. Muller &

15*

Bruyn, that in the third month after the laying of the corner-stone, on the 27th of September, 1867, the Synagogue was solemnly dedicated to the God of Israel by Rev. R. D'C. Lewin, and the congregation commenced regular worship in the new edifice. In January, 1868, Mr. Gertsman resigned the office of president and ceased officiating as lay reader. He was succeeded in the presidential chair by Mr. A. B. Weslow, and Mr. Rosenfeld, having given up his business in Florida and returned to Savannah, was elected the paid minister of the congregation. The congregation consists of about thirty members, nearly all of whom are natives of Poland. The "Minhag"* of the congregation is Polish, according to the orthodox form, although some few changes have been introduced. The congregation, though still young, promises to do well, and will doubtless progress as it grows older.

LUTHERAN CHURCH. There is little if any record remaining of the establishment of the Lutheran religion by the Salzburgers in Savannah. From the best information that can be gained, it appears that many members of the various colonies of Salzburgers who, during the period between 1736 and 1744, fled to Georgia to avoid persecution in their own land on account of their religion, remained in Savannah and formed the nucleus of a church organization about the year 1744. It was, however, for several years, regarded as a missionary ground, and the members were preached to at intervals by Revs. John Martin Bolzius and Israel Christian Gronau, of Ebenezer, and Rev. U. Driesler, of Frederica. A small church was built upon the site occupied by the present church, on the eastern side of Wright square. Revs. Rabenhorst and Wattman officiated in 1759. Rev. Mr. Bergman took charge of the church a short time before the Revolutionary war, during which the congregation, though much scattered, kept up its organization, and in 1787 the church was fully organized with a full board of elders and wardens. The services were conducted in the German language, of which the younger portion of the congregation were ignorant, a want of interest was manifested, the congregation decreased, and finally the church was closed. In 1824 Dr. Bachman, of Charleston, came over, and finding the families of Mr. Frederick Herb, Mr. Snider, Mr. Haupt, Mr. Spann, Mr. Gougle, Mr. Felt, Mrs. S. Cooper, Mrs. N. Weriman, and Mrs. L. Cooper, still attached to the faith, endeavored to resuscitate the congrega-

* Meaning custom—as in the form of ritual and pronunciation of the Hebrew.

tion, in which effort he was successful. Rev. Stephen A. Mealy came from Charleston in this year and took charge of the congregation, conducting the services in English. He remained until 1839, when he accepted a call to Philadelphia. Rev. N. Aldrich, of Charleston, became pastor in 1840. In 1843 the present building was erected, and was dedicated in the fall by the pastor, aided by Rev. Dr. Bachman. In 1850 Mr. Aldrich was succeeded by Rev. A. J. Karn, who remained until 1859. The church was closed until 1861, when Rev. J. Hawkins took charge, but he remained only eight or nine months. On his departure the church was again closed until the 1st of June, 1863, at which time the present pastor, Rev. D. M. Gilbert, took charge.

The church has about one hundred and thirty communicants, a fine Sunday-school numbering one hundred and seventy-five pupils under the superintendence of Mr. J. T. Thomas, and is in a flourishing condition. During the later periods, when the church was closed, the Sunday-school was in full operation, and devotional exercises were occasionally held.

PRESBYTERIAN: The first Presbyterian society in Savannah was organized about the year 1755, Rev. J. J. Zubly, D. D., pastor. The exact location of the first church is not known, but it was in Decker ward, and was destroyed by the fire of 1796. Another church was erected on the corner of York, President, and Whitaker streets, where a large livery stable now stands. The steeple of this church was blown down and the building injured during the gale of 1804. It was repaired and used until 1819, when it was taken down, and the congregation removed to the Independent Presbyterian church on Bull street, which is one of the most elegant and spacious houses of worship in the country. It was commenced in 1815 and completed in 1819, when it was dedicated by Rev. Dr. Henry Kollock; who died the following December. Rev. Dr. I. S. K. Axson is the present pastor of the church.

The elders since 1800 are: Thomas Young, John Gibbons, John Bolton, Jno. Hunter, Edward Stebbins, Geo. Harrell, Jno. Millen, John Cumming, Benjamin Burroughs, Moses Cleland, George W. Coe, John Lewis, George W. Anderson, James Smith, William Law, William Bee, G. B. Cumming, John Stoddard, G. B. Lamar, B. B. Hopkins.

The pastors who have had charge of the church since its organization are: Revs. John J. Zubly, D. D., Walter Monteith, Robert Smith, Samuel Clarkson, D. D., Henry Kollock, D. D., William D.

Snodgrass, D. D., Samuel B. How, D. D., Daniel Baker, Willard Preston, D. D., and I. S. K. Axson, D. D., the present pastor, who has been in charge since 1856.

Messrs. George W. Anderson, William Law, George B. Cumming, William H. Baker, John D. Hopkins, and Charles H. Olmstead are Elders, and Francis Sorrel, Anthony Porter, William Duncan, Chas. Green, and Charles F. Miller, Trustees.

There are three hundred and thirty-five communicants in this church, which has attached to it a fine Sunday-school, numbering one hundred and eighty-five scholars and teachers, under the superintendence of John D. Hopkins, Chas. H. Olmstead, Assistant Superintendent.

The FIRST PRESBYTERIAN CHURCH of Savannah was formally organized by the Presbytery of Georgia at a called meeting held in the old Baptist church on the 6th of June, 1827—the opening sermon being preached by the moderator, Rev. N. A. Pratt, of Darien. The number of members constituting the church then organized was about fifteen, the names of the following only being now known: James Cumming, Lowell Mason, Mrs. Gardiner, Miss Clifton, George G. Faries, W. King, Mrs. Coppee, Miss Burns, Edward Coppee, Miss M. Lavender, and Mrs. Faries.*

The elders of the church, chosen immediately after its organization, were: James Cumming, George G. Faries, E. Coppee, and L. Mason. Subsequent elders have been: W. Crabtree, J. J. Maxwell, B. E. Hand, John Ingersoll, E. J. Harden, Charles West, H. A. Crane, and J. F. Cann.

The first church was built upon the north side of Broughton, between Jefferson and Barnard streets, in 1833. Some time after the congregation left it, it was purchased by the Young Men's Christian association and removed to the northwest corner of Ann and Orange streets, where it was used for some time by the association, and was lately destroyed by fire. The present church edifice, situated on the east side of Monterey square, was commenced in 1856, but, owing to the loss of money and other circumstances beyond the control of the congregation, has not been completed. The work upon it, which was stopped at the commencement of the late war, will, it is thought, be soon recommenced, and a spacious and elegant building be erected. There are at present about eighty-five communicants. Judge E. J. Harden is superin-

---

* All of the original members, excepting Mr. King and Mrs. Coppee, are dead.

tendent of the Sunday-school, which numbers some sixty pupils. Rev. David H. Porter is pastor, and H. A. Crane, E. J. Harden, and A. M. Sloan, elders.

The pastors of the church, with an approximation of the dates of their ministry, are named as follows: Revs. Mr. Boggs, 1828; James C. Stiles, 1829; C. C. Jones, 1830; Mr. Holt, 1832; C. Blodget, 1832; J. L. Merrick, 1834; T. F. Scott, 1835; J. L. Jones, 1840—vacancy one year; B. M. Palmer, 1843--vacancy one year; J. B. Ross, 1853; John Jones, 1854; C. B. King, 1855; David H. Porter (the present pastor), 1855.

METHODISM. The first preacher sent to Savannah to propagate the doctrines of the Methodist Episcopal church was Rev. Beverly Allen, who came in 1785. He was followed by Revs. Hope Hull, Thomas Humphries, John Major, John Crawford, Phillip Mathews, Hezekiah Arnold, Wheeler Grisson, John Bonner, Jonathan Jackson, John Garvin, and Samuel Dunwoody, the latter of whom, in 1806, succeeded in organizing a Methodist society, and services were conducted in the houses of the Methodists. Rev. Hope Hull, for several years, preached in a cabinet-maker's shop belonging to Mr. Lowry. The society, in 1813, while under the pastoral charge of Rev. James Russell, commenced building a house of worship at the northeast corner of Lincoln and South Broad streets. It was completed in 1816, and dedicated by Rev. Lewis Myers. This edifice was called

The WESLEY CHAPEL. After being enlarged, remodeled, and repaired several times, the chapel was sold to Mr. W. B. Adams, in 1866, who converted it into private residences. A Sunday-school and lecture room was erected next to the church, but was destroyed by fire several years since. The congregation then purchased the building at the corner of Wayne and Drayton streets, formerly belonging to the German Lutheran congregation. The congregation is under the pastoral charge of Rev. D. D. Cox, and has one hundred and forty members. There is also a good Sunday-school, under the superintendence of Mr. J. H. Newman. The official members are: John Clements, A. C. Miller, W. H. Hubbard, W. H. Burrell, A. G. Bass; I. S. Anderson, Secretary of church meeting. The parsonage is located on the northeast corner of State and Habersham streets.

TRINITY CHURCH, a large and commodious brick edifice, and one of the handsomest churches in the city, is located on the west side of St. James square. It was commenced in 1848, during the pastorate of Rev. Dr. Alfred T. Mann, and completed in 1850, under the pastorate of Rev. J. E. Evans, and the following year was dedicated by Rev. Dr. Mann. The present membership numbers four hundred and twenty-six, Rev. G. G. N. McDonell pastor.

The stewards of the church are: R. D. Walker, John Houston, C. D. Rogers, James Lachlison, William M. Weaver, R. McIntire, C. A. Magill, J. R. Saussy, J. H. Newman, Benjamin Gammon. Rev. E. Heidt, elder, and George Allen, deacon, are local preachers; R. H. Tatem, Secretary of church meeting. The parsonage is located on the east side of Orleans square, and was bequeathed to the church by Mrs. Mary Ann Stafford in 1860, who also left about $20,000 in negro property for the poor of the church. The Sunday-school, with about three hundred and fifty scholars, is under the superintendence of Mr. C. D. Rogers.

The ANDREW CHAPEL was built for the colored people in 1845, through the energetic and persevering efforts of G. F. Pearce. For twenty years it was supplied with pastors by the Georgia Annual Conference, and had a large and flourishing membership. After the occupation of Savannah by General Sherman's army the great mass of the members united with the African M. E. Church, and have been supplied with pastors from that body ever since. The property is still held, however, by the trustees of the M. E. Church South, and a few of the old members continue faithful to their former church relations.

The trustees, who hold all property belonging to the M. E. Church South in Savannah, are: Robert D. Walker, E. Heidt, C. A. Magill, J. R. Saussy, Robert McIntire, Benjamin Gammon, C. D. Rogers, John Houston.

The names of all of the Methodist ministers ever stationed in Savannah are appended, many having been appointed here two or more times: Revs. Beverly Allen, Thomas Humphries, John Major, John Crawford, Phillip Mathews, Hope Hull, Hezekiah Arnold, Wheeler Grisson, John Bonner, Jonathan Jackson, John Garvin, Samuel Dunwoody, Jones H. Mallard, John McVean, Irving Cooper, James H. Kogler, Whitman C. Hill, James Russell, Henry Ross, Solomon Bryan, Wm. Capers (afterward Bishop), John Howard, James O. Andrew (afterward Bishop), George White, E. J. Fitzgerald, Thomas L. Wynn, George Hill, Charles Hardy, Elijah Sinclair, Benjamin Pope, Ignatius A. Few, George F. Pierce (afterward Bishop), Alexander Speer, James R. Evans, James Sewell. Miller H. White, James B. Jackson, Daniel Currie, Joseph Lewis,

Caleb W. Key, A. T. Mann, W. R. Branham, Robert Connor, Lovick Pierce, Wm. M. Crumley, Joshua S. Payne, Charles F. Cooper, Thomas H. Jordan, G. G. N. Macdonnell, Joseph S. Key, James M. Dickie, D. T. Holmes, Lewis B. Payne, W. H. Potter, L. G. R. Wiggings, W. P. Pledger, H. James, R. F. Breedlove, E. W. Speer, J. T. Norris, J. R. Caldwell, W. S. Baker, Walter Knox, Alexander M. Wynn, John W. Turner, John F. Ellerson, A. J. Corley, and D. D. Cox.

The BAPTIST CHURCH. About the year 1795 a Baptist house of worship was erected on Franklin square in this city, by different denominations both here and in South Carolina. The house, in an unfinished state, was rented for several years to the Presbyterian congregation, theirs having been destroyed by fire. In 1799, before the expiration of the lease, the Rev. Henry Holcombe, of Beaufort, S. C., was chosen pastor of the congregation, then consisting of different denominations. His salary was $2,000 per annum. The house of worship was dedicated on the 17th of April, 1800, and the church was dedicated on the 26th of November, in the same year. The Rev. Henry Holcombe was the pastor. A baptistery was placed in the church in 1800, and the first person baptised was a Mrs. Jones.

In the year 1795 the corporation of Savannah conveyed to the church, in fee simple, the lot (No. 19) on Franklin square, now occupied by the First African Baptist church. The following persons petitioned the legislature of Georgia for the charter of incorporation: Rev. Henry Holcombe, pastor; George Mosse, W. H. Matthers, John Rose, Elias Robert, Joseph Wiseman, Theodore Carlton, Joseph Davis, Isaac Sibley, and Wm. Parker.

Worship was continued on Franklin square until the year 1833, about which time the brick building on Chippewa square in Brown ward was finished. The building was enlarged in 1839, during the ministry of Rev. J. G. Binney. This building cost, in the aggregate, about $40,000, and is the one in which the church is now worshiping.

The following are the pastors of the church from its organization to the present time: Henry Holcombe, D. D., from 1799 to 1811; W. B. Johnson, D. D., 1811 to 1815; Benj. Scriven, 1815 to 1819; Jas. Sweat, 1819 to 1822; Thomas Meredith, 1822 to 1824; Henry O. Wyer, 1825 to 1834; Josiah S. Law, 1834 to 1835; Charles B. Jones, 1835 to 1836; J. G. Binney, 1836 to 1843; Henry O. Wyer, 1843 to 1845; Albert Williams, 1845 to 1847.

On the 4th of February, 1847, the church divided, Rev. Albert Williams, pastor. Thenceforward the two branches were popularly known as the First and Second Baptist churches, though the former never changed its corporate name. Those who constituted the Second Baptist church purchased the building then owned by the Unitarians on the southwest corner of Bull and York streets, where they continued to worship until the 6th of February, 1859, when they dissolved, and the reunion of the Baptists of Savannah occurred (after a separation of twelve years almost to a day) on the 6th of February, 1859.

Pastors of the First Church: Rev. Albert Williams, a part of 1847; Rev. Jos. T. Roberts, from 1847 to 1849; Rev. Thomas Rambaut, 1849 to 1855; Rev. J. B. Stiteler, 1855 to 1856; Rev. S. G. Daniel, 1856 to 1859.

Pastors of the Second Church: Rev. Henry O. Wyer, from 1847 to 1849; Rev. J. P. Tustin, 1849 to 1854; Rev. Henry O. Wyer, 1854 to 1855; Rev. M. Winston, 1855 to 1859.

Rev. Sylvanus Landrum (the present pastor) was called to Savannah in November, 1859, and settled with the church on the first day of the following month.

The deacons chosen on the 3d of March, 1859, were George W. Davis, James E. Hogg, O. M. Lillibridge, John W. Rabun, William F. Chaplin, and Isaac Brunner, four of whom are still living and in office.

In 1861 the church constructed the lecture and Sunday-school room in the basement of their building, and in 1862 purchased the Pastor's Home, on the corner of Jones and Drayton streets. During the year 1868, they purchased a lot (No. 19) in Loyd ward, corner of Barnard and Gwinnett streets, on which a mission church is to be built. The number of communicants is four hundred and fifteen.

The Sunday-school was organized on the 29th of April, 1827, and is finely arranged and admirably conducted. Mr. B. M. Zettler is superintendent and C. W. West secretary. The number of teachers is thirty-four; scholars, one hundred and eighty.

This church has no colored members. There are, however, three colored Baptist churches in the city. The first and second own good buildings and have a very large membership.

The government of the Savannah Baptist church, according to the practice of the denomination, is congregational, or independent. The church transacts her own business, executes her own discipline, and her decisions are final. She, however, holds an associated connection, for benevolent purposes, with the New Sunbury Association and with the Georgia Baptist Convention.

The CATHOLIC CHURCH. The Catholic religion was established in Savannah during the latter part of the last century. The first building was erected in Liberty square, and was taken down in 1838. There are about eight thousand five hundred members of this church in Savannah, which is divided into two parishes, St. John's and St. Patrick's. The former parish has about five thousand persons in it, who worship at the St. John's cathedral, a magnificent and capacious edifice, located on the east side of Drayton, at the corner of Perry street. Right Rev. Bishop A. Verot, and Rev. Fathers W. J. Hamilton and P. Whelan officiate in this parish. St. Patrick's parish was organized on the 6th of November, 1865. St. Patrick's church, in which the members of this parish, three thousand five hundred in number, worship has been used as a church edifice since the 8th of November, 1863. Very Rev. Peter Dufau, Vicar-General of the diocese, and Rev. Father C. C. Prendergast are in charge of this parish. The Sisters of Our Lady of Mercy have an extensive building situated on Liberty street, in which about two hundred females are instructed. A large number of them are orphans, under the care of the sisters, and a considerable number besides receive gratuitous instruction.

The PENFIELD MARINERS' CHURCH, located on Bay, near Lincoln street, was erected in 1831 with the money bequeathed for the purpose by Rev. Josiah Penfield.

The church is now under the management of the Savannah Port Society, which was organized on the 21st of November, 1843, "for the purpose of furnishing seamen with regular evangelical ministration of the Gospel, and such other religious instruction as may be found practicable." Messrs. John Lewis, W. W. Wash, Asa Holt, Robert M. Goodwin, John Ingersoll, Wm. Duncan, Robt. A. Lewis, Samuel Philbrick, S. Goodall, Benjamin Snider, J. R. Wilder, Thos. Clark, Michael Dillon, Charles Green, Rev. P. A. Strobel, Rev. E. F. Neufville, D. D., Rev. W. Preston, D. D., Captain William Crabtree, Joseph Felt, John Stoddard, Joseph George, Edward Wiley, Green Fleetwood, Edward Padelford, Joseph Cumming, John J. Maxwell, Mathew Hopkins, J. C. Dunning, and D. B. Williams, were among the founders.

The officers of the Society are: J. T. Thomas, President; John D. Hopkins, 1st Vice-President; C. D. Rogers, 2d Vice-President;

D. G. Purse, Treasurer; C. H. Olmstead, Recording Secretary; J. R. Saussy, Corresponding Secretary; Rev. Richard Webb, Chaplain.

BENEVOLENT SOCIETIES.

The societies in Savannah for the amelioration of the wants of the poor and distressed, and for the purpose of fostering fraternal relations, are numerous and flourishing. The records of the more prominent ones will be found below.

MASONIC. There is little else but tradition left regarding the origin of the first Lodge of the brethren of the "mystic tie" in Georgia. It is asserted that, early in 1733, a number of Masons under the leadership of General Oglethorpe, while at Sunbury, then a small settlement, organized, under a large oak tree,* a Lodge known afterward as the Savannah Lodge. This Lodge was chartered, in 1735, as Solomon's Lodge. After 1800, the Union, L'Esperance, Hiram, and Oglethorpe Lodges were organized. During the Morgan excitement all the Lodges, excepting Solomon's, were broken up. The first hall erected for the meetings of the Lodges is situated on President street, near St. James square. It is a long two-story frame building, now used as a private residence. The present hall, in which both the Masonic and Odd Fellows' Lodges meet, is an elegant brick structure situated on Broughton, at the northeast corner of Bull street.

The Solomon's Lodge, No. 1, A. F. M. (first known as the Savannah Lodge), was organized in 1733 and chartered in 1735. It is the oldest chartered Lodge in the United States. From 1776 to 1785, owing to the Revolutionary war, no meetings were held, and the records were lost. The officers are: P. M. John Nicolson, W. M.; Bros. J. Lachlison, S. W.; Bernard Brady, J. W.; J. C. Bruyn, Treas.; J. H. Estill, Sec.; John Oliver, S. D.; R. H. Lewis, J. D.; A. G. McArthur, Harmon A. Elkins, Stewards; De Witt Bruyn, Organist; John F. Herb, Tyler.

Georgia Chapter, No. 3, R. A. M., was established in 1818. The following are the officers: P. H. P. Richard T. Turner, M. E. H. P.; Companions R. J. Nunn, E. K.; Thomas Balentyne, E. S.; Rev. Sylvanus Landrum, Chaplain; S. P. Hamilton, C. H.; E. W. Marsh, P. S.; C. Heinsius, R. A. C.; J. H. Dews, M. 3d V.; Chas.

* A chair was made of a portion of this tree, and now ornaments the Masonic Lodge room in the Masonic Hall.

Pratt, M. 2d V.; J. C. McNulty, M. 1st V.; J. T. Thomas, Treas.; J. H. Estill, Sec.; M. M. Belisario, Sentinel.

Zerubbabel Lodge, No. 15, A. F. M., was chartered on the 5th of November, 1840. The officers are: P. M. L. M. Shafer, W. M.; Rev. Bro. R. D'C. Lewin, S. W.; Bro. Simon Hexter, J. W.; P. M. Alfred Haywood, Treas.; J. A. Sullivan, Sec.; Jas. Manning, S. D.; William D. Sullivan, J. D.; Jacob Belsinger, Moritz Kohl, J. Vetsburg, Stewards; I. H. Hollem, Organist; J. F. Herb, Tyler.

Clinton Lodge, No. 54, F. A. M., was chartered on the 27th of October, 1847. The officers are: P. M. C. F. Blancho, W. M.; P. M. M. M. Belisario, S. W.; Bros. John G. Blitch, J. W.; Wm. M. Davidson, Treas.; Levy E. Byck, Sec.; Lewis Kayton, S. D.; David Cockshutt, J. D.; John F. Herb, Tyler.

Ancient Landmark Lodge, No. 231, was chartered on the 15th of November, 1859. The following are the officers: Bros. Rufus E. Lester, W. M.; C. Heinsius, S. W.; E. W. Marsh, J. W.; C. M. Cunningham, Treas.; F. R. Sweat, Sec.; A. A. E. W. Barclay, S. D.; E. W. Marsh, J. D.; John F. Herb, Tyler.

Palestine Commandery, No. 7, K. T., was instituted on the 15th of April, 1867. The officers are: Theodore B. Marshall, E. C.; R. J. Nunn, G.; J. H. Gould, C. G.; E. W. S. Neff, Treas.; J. A. Roberts, P.; Rufus E. Lester, S. W.; S. P. Hamilton, J. W.; L. M. Shafer, R.; J. H. Estill, John H. Dew, Standard Bearers; John Nicolson, Warden; W. F. Parker, Sentinel.

The Union Society, whose achievements, to use the language of that gifted divine, Rev. Willard Preston, consist in rescuing the mind from the worst of despotisms—the cruel, degrading, withering grasp of ignorance; in training it to effort and to useful enterprise; in rescuing the child of misfortune from the deep and overwhelming, and but too often demoralizing and ruinous, depressions of poverty, and consequently relieving the widow from those burdens which often sink her into an untimely grave, was organized in 1750 by five gentlemen of five distinct religious denominations, having for their leading object the education of orphan children in indigent circumstances. Tradition has rescued from oblivion only three of the founders, viz: Benjamin Shefftall, Peter Tondee, and Richard Milledge. They called themselves the St. George's Society, and held their anniversaries on the 23d day of April, the calendar day of the canonization of the tutelar saint of England. The records were destroyed by the British when they evacuated the city in 1782, and very little is known of its early history. Among the rules was one requiring each member to contribute two pence weekly to carry out the object of the society; another, that any three of its members should hold regular meetings and celebrate its anniversaries. Twenty-eight years after its organization this rule saved the society from extinction. When Savannah was captured by the British in December, 1778, a large number of citizens (among them a number of members of the Union Society) and soldiers was placed on board of the prison-ships. A few days after, those of the prisoners who held office in the American army were sent, under parole, to Sunbury, a town forty miles distant, on the seacoast. Among these were four members of the society, Mordecai Shefftall, John Martin, John Stirk, and Josiah Powell, who were kept there three years, during which time they observed the meetings and kept the anniversaries of the society, at the first of which, held on the 23d of April, 1779, under a large oak tree,* the following resolution was adopted:

> By the unhappy fate of war, the members of the Union Society are some made captives and others drove from the State, and by one of the rules of said society it is ordered and resolved that so long as three members shall be together the Union Society shall exist; and there being now four members present who, being desirous as much as in them lies, notwithstanding they are CAPTIVES, to continue so laudable an institution, have come to the following resolve, to wit: To nominate and appoint officers for said society for the ensuing year as near and as agreeable to the rules of the society as they can recollect, the rules being lost or mislaid.

Josiah Powell was then elected president, Mordecai Shefftall vice-president, and John Martin secretary. An entertainment was then partaken of, a number of British officers who had furnished it participating. The sentiments given on the occasion equally express the noble and honorable feelings of both parties. The first, by a member of the society, was "The Union Society;" the second, by a British officer, "General George Washington," which was responded to with equal magnanimity by an American officer, "The King of Great Britain."

These gentlemen preserved the existence of the society, which in

---

* This tree was cut down some years after the meeting, and a beautiful box made of a portion of it. On the one hundredth anniversary (1850) of the society the box was presented to it by Mrs. Perla Sheftall Solomons, a descendant of one of the founders. The records and papers are now kept in this box, which is laid before the president upon every anniversary.

1786 was incorporated by the legislature of the State, with the title of the Union Society. In 1854 the Board of Managers of the society purchased one hundred and twenty-five acres of the Bethesda estate and erected buildings for the accommodation of the orphans under its charge, and removed them thither. There are now twenty-three boys under the charge of the society at Bethesda, which is under the superintendence of Rev. E. P. Brown.

The officers are: Abraham Minis, president; G. Moxley Sorrell, vice-president; John T. Thomas, secretary; D. G. Purse, treasurer; Edward Padelford, Andrew Low, Octavus Cohen, W. M. Wadley, C. H. Olmstead, F. W. Sims, R. Morgan, J. L. Villalonga, J. W. Lathrop, board of managers; Henry Bryan, E. J. Moses, stewards.

The following list embraces the presidents of the society so far as known. From 1750 to 1778 there is no record to show who filled the responsible position. In 1779 Josiah Powell was president, in 1786 Wm. Stephens, in 1790 Noble Wimberly Jones, from which year to the present the following have respectively held the position: Joseph Clay, Joseph Habersham, Wm. Stephens, George Jones, James P. Young, Mathew McAllister, Joseph Habersham, Charles Harris, General David B. Mitchell, Wm. B. Bulloch, Wm. Davies, J. McPherson Berrien, James Johnston, Dr. Moses Sheftall, John Hunter, Richard W. Habersham, Steele White, Thomas Polhill, John C. Nicoll, George W. Anderson, Francis Sorrell, Thomas Purse, Dr. R. D. Arnold, Solomon Cohen, Edward Padelford, Jos. S. Fay, Robert D. Walker, John M. Cooper, William M. Wadley, and Abraham Minis, the present president.

Robert Habersham, Esq., one of our oldest and most respected merchants, has been connected with the society sixty-two years, and attends all of the anniversaries.

St. Andrew's Society. This society, composed of the sons of old Scotia, was organized about 1790, its first president being General Lachlan McIntosh, with Sir George Houstoun as vice-president. During the war of 1812 the society seems to have died, as we find no notice of its meetings. About 1819 it was reorganized. In 1849 or 1850 the society purchased the lot on the southwest corner of Broughton and Jefferson streets, and erected upon it the present commodious hall. During the war the treasury became depleted, and the society was forced to dispose of the property. Its decaying fortunes have been revived of late, and the society is now in a flourishing condition. The officers are: John Cunningham, president; Robt Lachlison, first, and Wm. Rogers, second vice-president; E. A. McGill, secretary and treasurer; Alexander Irving and A. G. McArthur, stewards.

The MEDICAL SOCIETY. Upon petition, Noble Wimberly Jones, John Irvine, John Grimes, Lemuel Kollock, John Cumming, Jas. Ewell, Moses Sheftall, Joshua E. White, William Parker, Thomas Schley, George Jones, George Vinson Proctor, Henry Bourquin, Thomas Young, Jr., Peter Ward, William Cocke, James Glenn, and Nicholas S. Bayard, who had associated themselves under the above name "for improving the science of medicine and lessening the fatality induced by climate and incidental causes," were granted a charter by the legislature on the 12th of December, 1804.

At that period rice was cultivated on the low lands adjacent to the city, up to the very door-sills of the houses. This society early took the stand that, with our semi-tropical climate, there could be no worse nor more malignant incidental cause of disease than the stagnant water which remains on the rice fields exposed to an ardent summer sun and the subsequent exposure of the saturated soil when the water is drained off. As an effort toward the abatement of the evil, the society proposed a plan of dry culture providing that the lands then cultivated in rice, which obligates wet culture, should be cultivated solely in such products as necessitated drainage and dry culture. The prohibition of rice culture within a radius of one mile from the city limits was suggested as a remedial measure. But rice lands were valuable, and the owners of the land lying within the prescribed radius demurred to the project of putting their lands under dry culture when they were much more valuable under wet culture. The society persevered until, in 1817, the land owners came to terms, and, in consideration of the sum of forty dollars per acre, agreed to bind their lands for ever from being cultivated in wet culture. Savannah then had a population of about six thousand (about two fifths black) and paid two hundred thousand dollars to carry the project into effect. Well did Dr. R. D. Arnold remark, in a lecture delivered before the Medical Society in 1868, that this contribution was "a noble monument to the liberality of her citizens and a high tribute to the estimation in which our profession was held, when a sum so large in proportion to her population was freely given in support of what many still maintained was a mere theoretical idea. But it was a practical idea. Never were more decided results produced from any given cause."

The officers of the Society are: Juriah Harris, president; James B. Read, vice-president; Joseph C. Habersham, recording secretary; William M. Charters, corresponding secretary; John D. Fish, treasurer; R. J. Nunn, librarian.

The HIBERNIAN SOCIETY was organized on the 17th of March, 1812, by a number of Irish citizens. Among the first members of the society were John Cumming, Zachary Miller, John Dillon, David Bell, Isaac Minis, T. U. P. Charlton, and James Hunter. Of those who organized the society Mr. David Bell is the only one living. He is now eighty-nine years of age. He was one of the first members of the Savannah Volunteer Guards, and was to be found in the ranks of the company upon every parade day until a few years ago, when age and infirmity prevented. He was with the Guards on duty in the trenches around the city in 1812.

The society has the following officers: J. J. Kelly, president; John McMahon, vice-president; L. J. Guilmartin, treasurer; John R. Dillon, secretary; P. R. Shiels, standard bearer.

ODD FELLOWS. "Quotha, they are odd *enow* in excellence," says an odd play, and this is confirmed by the six societies in Savannah which are day by day developing the holy principles of the order.

The Oglethorpe Lodge was instituted in 1842. The officers are: D. Ferguson, N. G.; F. Kreiger, V. G.; C. Gross, P. and R. S.; J. Oliver, T.

Live Oak Lodge, No. 3, was instituted in 1843. The following are the officers: C. E. Wakefield, N. G.; John Cooper, V. G.; John F. Herb, R. and P. G.; William E. White, T.

Magnolia Encampment was instituted in 1845. The officers are: F. D. Jordan, G. P.; J. F. Herb, S.; J. Neal, S. W.; T. H. Bolshaw, J. W.; C. E. Wakefield, H. P.

De Kalb Lodge was instituted in 1845. The officers are: C. W. West, N. G.; B. T. Cole, V. G.; W. S. Hubbard, P. and R. S.

Wildney Degree Lodge was instituted in 1867. The officers are: John Neill, H. P.; T. H. Bolshaw, D. H. P.; Benjamin Cole, Jr., S.; C. E. Wakefield, T.

Haupt Lodge, No. 57, was instituted on the 14th of January, 1869. The officers are: C. F. Blancho, N. G.; Thomas H. Laird, V. G.; T. W. McNish, P. and R. S.; Jos. B. Sibley, Treasurer.

The IRISH UNION SOCIETY was organized on the 17th of March, 1847, having for its object the amelioration of the condition of the fellow countrymen of its members. The first officers were John Murphy, president, and Philip Kean, vice-president; John Everard, treasurer; Martin Duggan, secretary; Thomas Forde, standard bearer. The officers now are: Judge Dominick A. O'Byrne, president; Andrew Flatley, vice-president; William J. Flynn, secretary; John O'Connell, standard bearer.

The HEBREW BENEVOLENT SOCIETY. The initiatory proceedings for the organization of this society took place on the evening of September 22d, 1851, at the house of Rudolph Einstein, Esq., where, at a meeting of Israelites specially convened for the purpose and presided over by Abraham Einstein, Esq., the plans for the establishment of the proposed society were discussed and committees appointed to prepare the necessary constitution and enlist the sympathies of the Israelites in the project. Two evenings afterward a large and influential meeting was held at the house of Abraham Einstein, Solomon Cohen presiding as chairman, on which occasion the society was established, eighty-one gentlemen having enrolled their names as members. Solomon Cohen was elected president of the society, whose object is to minister to the necessities of the indigent. In addition to the regular officers, a committee of four is appointed, who possess supervisory power over the relief distributed.

The officers are as follows: Abraham Epstein, president; Solomon Gardner, vice-president; S. H. Eckman, treasurer; L. W. Stern, secretary; A. J. Brady, E. Ehrlich, S. E. Byck, trustees. The charity committee consists of Rev. R. D'C. Lewin, chairman; L. Lilienthal and J. M. Solomons.

The LADIES' GERMAN BENEVOLENT SOCIETY was founded in 1853. Its object is identical with that of the Hebrew Benevolent Society. The meetings of the society are held quarterly. The officers are: Mrs. Joseph Lippman, president; Mrs. S. H. Eckman, treasurer; Mrs. M. Loewenthal, secretary.

The HARMONIE CLUB. The history of this club dates back to 1865. It was instituted for social and mental improvement, and made considerable progress under its first president, Mr. Wolf. Renting St. Andrew's Hall for their meetings, the members of the club are enabled to give those pleasant balls and social gatherings which add so much to the winter amusements of the city. The officers are: M. Loewenthal, president; L. Elsinger, vice-president; S. Gerstman, treasurer; J. Vetsburg, secretary.

The YOUNG MEN'S LIBRARY ASSOCIATION was organized on the 24th of June, 1866, under the auspices of Rev. A. M. Wynn, pastor of Trinity Methodist church, and was composed only of young men connected with that church. On the 15th of June, 1868, it was reorganized, and thrown open to the young men of all denominations. There are one hundred members connected with the association, and about four hundred volumes in the library. The officers are: General George P. Harrison, president; Rev. G. G. N. McDonell, vice-president; F. L. Hale, secretary and treasurer; J. C. Mather, librarian.

The St. George's Society, organized on the 18th of April, 1868, is composed entirely of Englishmen or their descendants, with the following officers: W. T. Smith (British Consul), president; John Oliver, vice-president; W. C. Cosens, secretary; Alfred Haywood, treasurer.

Joseph Lodge, No. 76, I. O. B. B., was organized on the 3d of June, 1866, for the advancement of the interests of the Jewish religion among its followers and for benevolent purposes. The officers are: Simon E. Byck, president; Isaac S. Davidson, vice-president; Isaac S. Cohen, secretary; Solomon Gardner, treasurer; Rev. R. D'C. Lewin, lecturer; Philip Dzialynski, assistant monitor; Jacob Cohen, warden; Isaac Cohen, guardian.

NEWSPAPERS.

The Georgia Gazette was started in Savannah on the 7th of April, 1763, by Mr. James Johnson, making the eighth newspaper then in the Colonies. This paper flourished as a weekly until 1799, when it was suspended. In the days of this newspaper there was no "local" column, and the only matters published concerning the city affairs were the marriages, deaths, and arrivals of vessels. Intercourse between Savannah and Charleston, in those days, was frequent. The Charleston editor obtained from the citizens of Savannah all information connected with the "Forest City," and published it. This the Georgia Gazette would copy in its next issue, about two weeks afterward. In the same way did the Savannah paper get its information concerning matters in Charleston.

The Savannah Republican. On the 1st of January, 1802, the first number of "The Georgia Republican," a semi-weekly paper, issued Tuesday and Friday, made its appearance in Savannah, Ga., edited and owned by John F. Everett, under which name it continued until March 10, 1807, when Jno. J. Evans became interested, under the firm name of Everett & Evans. The publication was then changed to a tri-weekly afternoon edition, issued Tuesdays, Thursdays, and Saturdays, under the name of "The Republican and Savannah Evening Ledger." It was published by Everett & Evans until the 28th of June, 1810, when John J. Evans continued it alone—no announcement being made of the withdrawal of Mr. Everett—until the 1st of January, 1814, when Mr. Frederick S. Fell became the editor and proprietor—the motto of the paper "Free Trade and no Impressment."

On the 11th of March, 1817, Mr. A. McIntyre was taken as a copartner into the concern, under the firm name of F. S. Fell & Co.

On the 17th of October, 1817, the paper was changed to a daily, and continued as such during the fall and winter months, and returned, during the summer, to tri-weekly issues. During the winter, besides a daily, a tri-weekly was also issued, which last publication was for country subscribers. The country, or tri-weekly paper, contained all the matter of the daily, besides the new advertisements. In both editions the Savannah market appeared weekly. Motto of the paper, "Truth without Fear." It contained a large amount of reading matter, and the advertising columns were well patronized. In order to accommodate its advertising patrons, it was necessary to issue, very often, a supplemental sheet.

On the 30th of October, a fortnight after the paper was changed from tri-weekly to daily, it was considerably enlarged. The pages of the former contained but four columns, while those of the latter had five columns, printed on a sheet twenty-four by thirty inches. The price of the daily, $8; tri-weekly, $6 per annum—payable in advance. The enlargement of the paper did not do away with the necessity of issuing the regular supplemental sheets for advertisements, so encouraging was that branch of patronage.

On the 10th of February, 1818, the Republican and Ledger commenced carrying on the job printing business in connection with the paper, having "employed one hand and a press" for this branch of their business, exclusively.

In June, 1818, F. S. Fell again published the paper alone—the firm name of F. S. Fell & Co. having been discontinued.

On the 21st of August, 1821, James G. Greenhow became associated with F. S. Fell, under the firm name of Fell & Greenhow, which continued until March 30th, 1822, when the copartnership was dissolved and Mr. Fell became again sole proprietor and editor.

On the 29th of May, 1830, Emanuel DeLaMotta took an interest with Mr. Fell, under the firm name of Fell & DeLaMotta, which copartnership was dissolved on the 10th of October, 1831, by the death, after a protracted illness, of Mr. Fell. This was the first death that occurred to a proprietor of the paper while in the active discharge of his duties. Mr. Fell filled the position of editor and publisher of the Republican seventeen years. The columns of the paper were clad in deep mourning for three consecutive issues after his death.

Mr. DeLaMotta continued the publication of the Republican alone from this date until June 1st, 1837, when Mr. I. Cleland became interested with him, under the copartnership name of DeLaMotta & Cleland, which remained in existence until the 11th of June, 1839, when Mr. DeLaMotta withdrew. From this date until February 15, 1840, Mr. Cleland was the sole publisher, when he became associated with Mr. William Hogan, under the firm name of Cleland & Hogan. This last copartnership only lasted till the 6th of July of the same year, when Mr. Cleland sold out his interest to Mr. Charles Davis, former proprietor of the Brunswick Advocate. Hogan & Davis was the firm name. Motto of the paper: "Union of the Whigs for the sake of the Union." It then became an active advocate of Whig principles, and was immediately changed from an afternoon to a morning issue, and continued daily throughout the year, at $10 per annum.

On the 12th of August, 1840 (the same year), Mr. Hogan disposed of his interest to Joseph L. Locke—firm name Locke & Davis—Mr. Locke senior editor and Mr. Davis commercial editor and business director. On the 26th of the following October the paper was again enlarged—seven columns to the page and length in proportion. This firm continued until the 30th of June, 1847, when, Mr. Davis' health becoming impaired, necessarily requiring a change of climate, he sold his interest to Mr. Francis J. Winter. Mr. Winter only survived until the following March (1848), being the second proprietor who died while in possession of an interest in the concern.

The firm name of Locke & Winter continued, after the death of Mr. Winter, until June 1st, 1848, when Mr. Locke became sole proprietor, and on the 17th of the following month (July) Mr. P. W. Alexander took position as associate editor with Mr. Locke—the paper published by J. L. Locke.

January 22d, 1849, A. K. Moore acquired an interest in the Republican and became its business manager.

July 1st, 1851, the price of subscription was reduced from $10 to $8 per annum.

On the 1st of January, 1853, Mr. Locke retired from the Repubcan, having sold out his interest to his editorial associate, P. W Alexander, who, in connection with Mr. Moore, published it under the firm name of P. W. Alexander & Co. This copartnership continued until the 19th of June, 1855, when Mr. Moore was announced as having retired, and Mr. James R. Sneed became a copartner with Mr. Alexander, under the firm name of Alexander & Sneed. Though Mr. Sneed became interested in the paper from this date, he did not arrive in Savannah, from Washington, Wilkes county, Ga., until the 21st of August, following, and on the 22d his salutatory appeared, from which time he entered upon the active duties of associate editor with Mr. Alexander.

On the 1st of July, 1856, Mr. Alexander withdrew from the Republican. His interest, being two thirds, was sold to Mr. James R. Sneed and Mr. F. W. Sims, so as to make them equal owners, and the firm name became that of Sneed & Sims—Mr. Sneed as the principal editor and Mr. Sims commercial editor and business manager. This firm continued until the 1st of January, 1858, when Mr. Sneed disposed of his interest to his copartner, Mr. Sims, but continued as its editor until the capture of Savannah by General Sherman and his army.

On the 29th of December, 1864, John E. Hayes, war correspondent of the New York Tribune, who had been following the army of General Sherman, took possession of the Republican office and its contents, by military authority, to publish a paper in the interest of the Federal government. He continued in the position of its editor and proprietor up to the time of his death, which occurred suddenly on the 16th day of September, 1868.

Frequent efforts were made by Mr. Sims (who had served in the Confederate armies) to reclaim his office, but unsuccessfully. A compromise was at length agreed upon, and his claim submitted to arbitration, when Mr. Sims was awarded about one fourth of its original cost.

During the administration of Mr. Hayes, the paper was in the interest of the Republican party up to within a short time of his death, when it became a conservative sheet.

At the death of Mr. Hayes the office went into the hands of his administrator, and was sold at public outcry on the 6th day of October, 1868, when Mr. James R. Sneed, its former editor and proprietor, by whom it is now (January, 1869) owned and conducted, became the purchaser.

Among the associate editors of the Republican since 1845, the following gentlemen, each for a time, rendered services on the paper: Messrs. S. T. Chapman, Edwin DeLeon, Thomas H. Harden, and Thomas W. Lane. For awhile before his last illness, the late Dr. William A. Caruthers, a distinguished writer of his time, was one of its regular contributors, and the eloquence of his style and diction gave additional interest to the columns of the paper.

In the fall of 1845 Mr. Locke made a tour of Europe, and during his sojourn there interested the readers of the Republican with a series of highly interesting and edifying letters, giving glowing and graphic descriptions of each point he visited. This was his first visit across the Atlantic while connected with the paper. He subsequently paid the continent another visit and resumed his correspondence.

In politics, the Republican, throughout its history, has been devoted to conservative views. For the first twenty years of its existence, it took no very active part in the political struggles of the times, though its sympathies were with the then Republican, or Jeffersonian party. It was an ardent advocate of Troup when the party that clustered around him in the State were opposed by Clarke and his political friends, and it warmly sustained General Jackson for the Presidency in the celebrated contest of 1828. During the second year of Jackson's administration, alarmed by what it considered the usurpations and abuses of the Executive, it gave the weight of its influence to the States' Rights party, and subsequently to the Whigs, with whom it acted throughout the existence of that organization, though it declined to support General Scott, its nominee, for the Presidency. During the contests that resulted in the late civil war between the States, the views of the Republican were conservative. It opposed the secession of the Southern States as unjustified by any grievance then in existence—that it would surely result in a terrible and disastrous war, for which we were wholly unprepared, and that our true policy was to fight our battles in the Union and under the constitution, at least until the wrongs of our section should become intolerable. When the Convention of Georgia took the State out of the Union, the Republican allied itself with her destiny, and was among the foremost in giving encouragement to the arms and councils of the Southern Confederacy. At the fall of the city, as previously stated, the paper fell into new and strange hands, and for several years was devoted to the conquerors. Restored to the hands of the gentleman who controlled its columns during the war and for five years preceding, it is now battling with zeal for the restoration of harmony and the Union under the Constitution.

The SAVANNAH GEORGIAN commenced publication on the 25th of November, 1818, by Dr. John Harney. About two years after, he sold the paper and material to I. K. Tefft and Henry Friend, who shortly afterward sold it to George Robertson. He subsequently associated with him his brother, William Robertson. The latter purchased the interest of his brother (George R.) and conducted the paper until the close of the year 1832, when it was disposed of to Dr. R. D. Arnold and William H. Bulloch, who were the joint editors and proprietors until 1835, when Mr. Bulloch purchased Dr. A.'s interest in the paper, and in 1849 conveyed it to Henry R. Jackson and Phillip J. Punch, who subsequently admitted S. S. Sibley as a partner. When General Jackson retired R. B. Hilton, of Florida, united himself with Messrs. Punch & Sibley. After several years connection with the paper Colonel Sibley left it, and it was published by Punch & Hilton; Punch, Hilton & Ganahl; P. J. Punch & Co.; Wright & Register; J. G. Wright & Co.; and perhaps one or two others, until the Journal and Courier was merged with it, when it came under the control of Albert R. Lamar, who revived its waning fortunes for a time, but the changes and unfortunate management had so weakened the paper that it was impossible to regain its ancient standing, and in 1859 its publication was suspended, and has never since been resumed.

The SAVANNAH MUSEUM was started about 1820, as a daily, by Keppel & Bartlett. It was in existence several years—how many, is not definitely known.

The SAVANNAH MORNING NEWS. The publication of this paper was commenced on the 15th day of January, 1850, by John M. Cooper, publisher, and W. T. Thompson, editor. At that time there were but two daily papers in Savannah—the Republican and the Georgian, both political journals—the first the organ of the Whig and the latter of the Democratic party of the State. The establishment of the News was projected with a view to furnish Savannah, then the rapidly thriving commercial emporium of the State, with an independent news and commercial medium, as nearly upon the plan of the cheap dailies of the Northern cities as was practicable. To furnish a medium for the dissemination of political truth, unbiased by party affiliation and control, was an object not secondary to the general purposes of the proprietors. The News, keeping aloof from party politics, took a decided position on the great sectional questions of the day, maintaining that the perpetuity of the Union depended upon a strict observance of the compromises and guarantees of the constitution, as affecting the rights and sovereign character of the States. To this position the paper steadfastly adhered to the close of the struggle which verified its prediction. The News was originally published on a sheet very little more than half its present dimensions, at four dollars per annum, or twelve and a half cents per week, payable to the carriers.

In the nineteen years of its existence, the Morning News has several times changed proprietors, while its present editor, Colonel W. T. Thompson, has been its principal editor all that time, except from the fall of Savannah in December, 1864, to August, 1865, when he resumed his identification with the paper as associate editor, with Mr. S. W. Mason, its late proprietor.

The following gentlemen have at different periods been editorially associated with the Savannah Morning News: Major T. A. Burke (now of Macon), Mr. E. O. Withington (at one time also a part proprietor), J. N. Cardoza, Esq., Dr. James S. Jones, and S. W. Mason, Esq., deceased.

From the commencement of its publication, in 1850, to March, 1855, Mr. John M. Cooper was proprietor, though for a short time other parties were associated with him as publishers. From March, 1855, to July, 1858, Colonel Thompson was both proprietor and editor—Mr. Withington being his partner and associate editor for a part of the time. In July, 1858, Messrs. Blois and Desvergers became the proprietors of the News, which was, in October of the same year, purchased entire by Mr. T. Blois, by whom, with Mr. Cooper and Colonel Aaron Wilbur—the latter of whom purchased an interest a few months before the fall of Savannah—as partners, the paper was continued to be published until the occupation of the city by the Federal troops.

Upon the occupation of the city the News establishment was taken possession of by Mr. John E. Hayes, who carried all the moveable material to the Republican office, of which he had also taken possession. Mr. Mason finally getting possession of the News office, brought from Hilton Head the materials with which he had published a small paper called the Palmetto Herald. With this, and the presses remaining in the News office, he commenced the publication of the Savannah Herald, subsequently settling the claims of the previous proprietors of the News establishment, which were submitted to arbitration. The name of the paper was then changed to the Daily News and Herald.

The present proprietor, Mr. J. H. Estill, originally purchased a part interest in the Morning News and entered upon the management of its business and mechanical department in July, 1867. A year afterward Mr. Estill purchased Mr. Mason's interest and resumed the original name of the paper, Savannah Morning News.

The EVENING JOURNAL was started by J. B. Cubbedge in 1851. The following year the Savannah Daily Courier was started by S. T. Chapman, and the Evening Mirror by W. B. Harrison. The Mirror was suspended soon after its birth, and the Journal and Courier were merged into one paper, known as the Journal and Courier, and published by Messrs. Chapman & Cubbedge until the death of the former, in 1854, when the paper was suspended for a short time, until it was purchased by Mr. R. B. Hilton. This paper was merged into the Georgian about 1857, and the consolidated papers published under the name of the Georgian and Journal.

The EVENING EXPRESS was started in 1859, by Ambrose Spencer and J. H. Estill. In 1860 its publication was suspended.

The DAILY ADVERTISER. This paper was started in September, 1865, as a free circulating journal (the first in the South) by Messrs. Theodore Hamilton and M. J. Divine, the former one of the managers of the Savannah theatre, and the latter a practical printer. They made arrangements with Mr. George N. Nichols for the use of his material. After running the paper a week these gentlemen disposed of their interest to Mr. Nichols, Mr. Hamilton retiring and Mr. Divine remaining as foreman. In the course of the following two months it was twice enlarged, and Mr. E. O. Withington, who had been connected with the paper since its first issue, was installed as editor. After a career of some six months more, a copartnership was formed between Messrs. Withington, Divine, and George S. Gray, under the firm name of E. O. Withington & Co., under which the paper continued, still as a free journal, until January 1st, 1868, when it was enlarged, changed to a subscription paper, and S. Yates Levy, Esq., engaged as editor-in-chief. Under his able editorial management the Advertiser at once took rank with the leading journals of the State. Mr. L. was a vigorous and fearless writer, pointing out and condemning abuses wherever discovered. So keen were some of his remarks upon the tyrannical actions of the military that an order was sent from Gen. Meade to either suppress the paper or moderate the tone of its editorials. Soon after Mr. Levy was obliged, by military pressure, to retire from the editorial chair.

In the latter part of May arrangements were made by the managers to sell out the paper to a gentleman of much experience in newspaper life. In order to perfect the changes necessary, it was determined to suspend for a month; but before the expiration of that time the gentleman declined to consummate the arrangement.

Nothing further was done until November, when Messrs. Edward L. Beard and George G. Kimball, formerly connected with the Savannah Republican, took charge of the paper, and are now running it again as a free journal.

The Mercantile Index was started in 1865, by George H. Johnstone, Jr., and E. M. Purse, but was suspended after an existence of about six months.

SUBURBAN RESORTS.

Savannah is fortunate in her suburban relations. Bethesda, Thunderbolt, White Bluff, Bonaventure, and Jasper Spring, all of easy access from the city, present attractions to the tourist that amply repay a visit. Independent of their historical associations, their intrinsic beauty is their best commendation.

Bethesda, signifying a "House of Mercy," is situated about ten miles from Savannah, where there is an orphan-house under the auspices of the Union Society.

In 1737 Rev. Geo. Whitfield, whose popularity in England was so great that those who came to hear him preach sometimes numbered twenty thousand, and many who were forced to remain outside prayed only for a sight of "his blessed face," turned his back on fame and fortune and sought what was then the wilds of Georgia, believing that God was calling him to undertake the mission. He labored among the inhabitants with unwonted zeal, and observing that the poverty of the inhabitants imperatively demanded the establishment of an orphan-house, suggested to him originally by Rev. Charles Wesley, he labored long and diligently in the furtherance of his plan, meeting a ready and willing assistant in James Habersham, who had accompanied him to Georgia, and whom he called his "beloved fellow-traveler." To further the object, Whitfield returned to England and secured from the Trustees "five hundred acres of any vacant land which he should select." The people of England to whom he preached gave with liberal hands to the charity. On his return to Savannah the ground was selected—the present ground forming part of it—by Mr. Habersham, and on the 25th of March, 1740, Whitfield "laid with his own hands the first brick of this great house, which he called Bethesda." This charity was never out of the mind of Whitfield, and with a parent's ardor and abiding love he clung to it and labored for it. For thirty years this labor lasted, and in the very year of his death, 1770, when his strength had yielded and his life was fast ebbing away, he projected a plan of a college to be added to the House of Mercy, and preached in the chapel there before the Governor, Council, and Assembly, whom he had invited hither to secure their co-operation.

Selina, Countess of Huntingdon, born and reared amid the splendor of high rank, beautiful, accomplished, and talented, became a convert to Methodism. She met Whitfield, and having her sympathies enlisted in his noble work, gave her money, her counsel, and her countenance to him. The Orphan-House became her work almost as much as his, and when he died his will was found to contain a clause devising Bethesda to her, "and in case she should be called upon to enter upon her glorious rest before my decease, to Hon. James Habersham, a merchant of Savannah." She did not falter when this responsibility was thrust upon her, but did all that could be done, but its sun of prosperity had set in Whitfield's grave. The buildings were struck by lightning and consumed. They were rebuilt, but disaster followed disaster, and in 1782 the Royal troops, previous to their evacuation of the city, destroyed everything of value. Lady Huntingdon, until her death, which occurred in 1791, labored with indomitable perseverance and christian zeal to forward the interests of Bethesda, but with comparatively little success. At her death the school was discontinued, and the State government reclaimed it and committed its management to a Board of Trustees. The Board took no active steps toward completing the buildings, nor other necessary measures for the organization of the school, until 1801. The property was rebuilt and the school reorganized, but in 1805 a fire destroyed one of the wings so that it could not be repaired, and a hurricane destroyed the out-buildings. The Trustees being unable to rebuild, in 1808 they advised the legislature to dispose of the property and distribute the proceeds among the benevolent institutions of Savannah. Accordingly, on the 12th of March, 1809, the property was sold.

In the year 1854 the Board of Managers of the Union Society, an institution similar in purposes and operations to Bethesda, purchased one hundred and twenty-five acres of the ancient Bethesda estate, which included the original locality of the Whitfield Orphan-House. They at once erected suitable buildings, and in January, 1855, removed the boys under their charge from Savannah to this place. This was purchased by the Union Society at a higher price than that at which some other places might have been obtained, and perhaps above its market value, from the fact that upward of a century ago it had been consecrated to the same noble purpose.

BONAVENTURE, whose melancholy beauty challenges comparison with any spot of similar magnitude in the country, is situated about four miles from Savannah. Originally a cemetery, it contains many fine specimens of sepultural architecture, which time has invested with hallowed remembrances. Numerous lofty oaks lend their grateful shade to the last resting-places of the silent dead, and the character of the foliage presents a unique and almost indescribable appearance, draped as it is with weeping festoons of moss, whose luxuriant growth makes the shade impenetrable to the sun's rays. Nature and the wise neglect of man have made it a peerless combination of the sublime and picturesque.

THUNDERBOLT, another of those "lungs of the city" which render a residence in Savannah peculiarly agreeable, is a collection of some two or three hotels and a score or so of private residences, pleasantly situated upon the banks of the river to which the village has given its name. Distant about five miles southeast of the city, it is noted more for the splendid drive, of which it is the terminus, than for any intrinsic natural beauty. The Savannah race-track, which is contiguous, materially enhances the popularity of the place, and the patrons of the turf find ample opportunity during the racing season to test the qualities of their stock. Its name, in the quaint literalness of General Oglethorpe's account of Carolina and Georgia, is derived "from the fall of a thunderbolt," and he adds that "a spring thereupon arose in that place, which still smells of the bolt."

WHITE BLUFF, situated on the Vernon river, about ten miles from the city, is also a popular place of resort, and the route to it during fine weather is marked by a train of equipages that would do credit to a city of metropolitan standing. The accommodations for visitors at present are limited to two hotels, but with the rapid advancement of Savannah others will doubtless be built. A number of summer residences impart an air of importance to this well-known locality. It is deficient in historical reminiscence, and therefore little can be said on this subject. A small Dutch settlement occupied the Bluff in 1740.

JASPER SPRING, situated on the Augusta road, two miles from Savannah, is noted as being the scene of the bold exploit of Sergeants Jasper and Newton previous to the siege of Savannah. Sergeant Jasper, after his exploit at Fort Moultrie, was granted a roving commission by Colonel Moultrie, commanding the 2d South Carolina regiment, with the privilege of selecting such men as he pleased. The scouts of Jasper were frequent and productive of much good, on account of the information he brought.* On one occasion he met, near Ebenezer, a lady named Mrs. Jones, who was in great distress about her husband. He had taken the oath of allegiance to the British government; afterward joined the American army and was captured by the British, who determined to hang him, with others who were to be carried to Savannah for that purpose the next morning. She appealed to Jasper to rescue him. He was moved by her distress, and promised to do what he could. Sergeant Newton was near by and Jasper consulted him, but they could arrange no plan. They, however, determined to follow the guard the next day, and take advantage of any opportunity that might be offered. Early in the morning a guard, consisting of a sergeant, a corporal, and eight men, started with the prisoners in irons. The wives and children of two or three of the prisoners followed. Jasper and Newton also followed closely, and upon coming near the spring, got ahead of the party and hid in the bushes, thinking that the guard would halt to get water, and a a chance to rescue the prisoners be presented. The guard came up and halted on the roadside. The arms were stacked and two men placed on guard over them and the prisoners near by. The rest of the guard then went to the spring. Jasper and Newton crept up to the two sentinels, shot them down, seized the stack of muskets, and called upon the rest of the astonished guard to surrender. A moment's reflection showed that they were completely at the mercy of the two determined men, and a surrender was made. The irons were knocked off of the prisoners and placed upon the soldiers, who were then conducted to the American camp at Purysburgh.

* Jasper at one time came into Savannah and spent several days without discovery, during which time he collected valuable information concerning the numbers and position of the British forces and furnished it to General Lincoln.

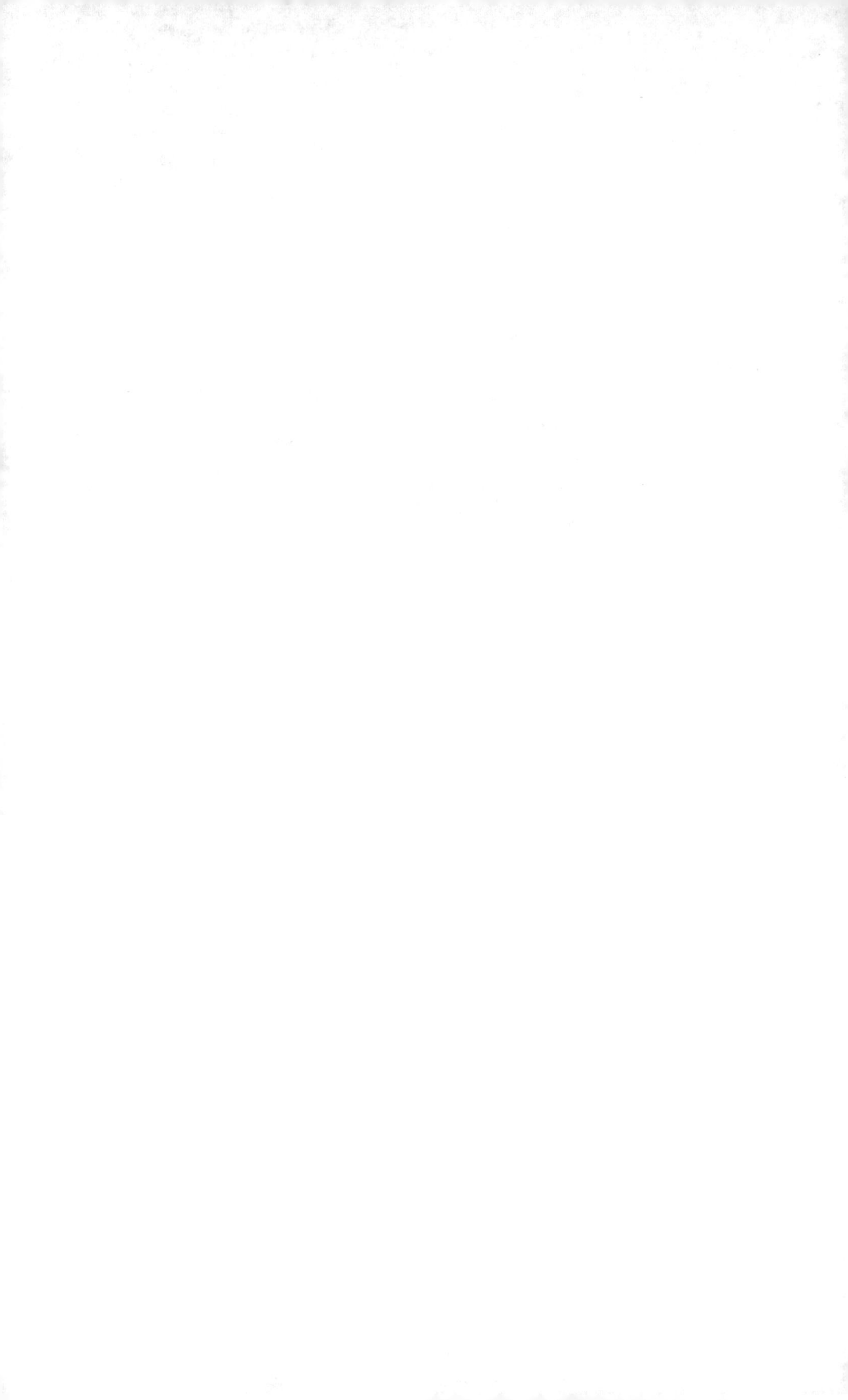

www.ingramcontent.com/pod-product-compliance
Lightning Source LLC
LaVergne TN
LVHW011203110826
845150LV00006B/1309

* 9 7 8 1 4 2 5 5 1 8 4 9 3 *